The Breast Health Checklist

The Breast Health Checklist

Simple Checklists to Keep You Organized,
Informed & In Control of Your Breast Care

Rand J. Stack, MD

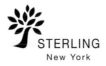

STERLING
New York

STERLING
New York

An Imprint of Sterling Publishing Co., Inc.
1166 Avenue of the Americas
New York, NY 10036

ISBN 978-1-4549-2580-4

Library of Congress Cataloging-in-Publication Data

Names: Stack, Rand J., author.
Title: The breast health checklist : simple checklists to keep you organized
  & informed in managing & treating breast cancer / Rand J. Stack, MD.
Description: New York, NY : Sterling, [2018] | Includes bibliographical
  references and index.
Identifiers: LCCN 2018000118 | ISBN 9781454925804 (paperback)
Subjects: LCSH: Breast--Cancer--Prevention. | Breast--Cancer--Risk factors. |
  Breast--Cancer--Treatment. | Breast--Care and hygiene. | BISAC: HEALTH &
  FITNESS / Diseases / Cancer. | HEALTH & FITNESS / Breastfeeding. | HEALTH
  & FITNESS / Women's Health.
Classification: LCC RC280.B8 S723 2018 | DDC 616.99/449052--dc23
LC record available at https://lccn.loc.gov/2018000118

Distributed in Canada by Sterling Publishing Co., Inc.
C/o Canadian Manda Group, 664 Annette Street
Toronto, Ontario M6S 2C8, Canada
Distributed in the United Kingdom by GMC Distribution Services
Castle Place, 166 High Street, Lewes, East Sussex BN7 1XU, England
Distributed in Australia by NewSouth Books
45 Beach Street, Coogee NSW 2034, Australia

For information about custom editions, special sales, and premium and corporate purchases,
please contact Sterling Special Sales at 800-805-5489 or specialsales@sterlingpublishing.com.

Manufactured in China

2 4 6 8 10 9 7 5 3 1

sterlingpublishing.com

Cover design by Elizabeth Mihaltse Lindy

For Picture Credits, see page 195

THIS BOOK IS DEDICATED TO
MY PARENTS, ELLY AND JERRY; MY WIFE, CONNIE;
AND MY THREE CHILDREN, DEBORAH, WALTER, AND DAVID.

Contents

The Checklists

Breast Health Diary

Why a Book of Checklists?

I WROTE THIS BOOK AS A PHYSICIAN SPECIALIZING IN MAMMOGRAPHY, breast imaging, and breast biopsy. Over the years, I have met with countless patients to explain the results of their mammograms. Every week, I speak to women who have come to my office for a routine mammogram and are stunned to learn that I found an abnormality that requires a breast biopsy. In my daily practice, I see how frightening and upsetting it can be to have breast health suddenly become the most important priority in a woman's mind.

If you are diagnosed with breast cancer, this easy-to-understand book will guide you step by step through your diagnosis and treatment. The checklists you'll find here are valuable tools to help you organize your thoughts, decide which questions need to be asked, and formulate a plan for moving forward with an effective strategy to overcome a potentially overwhelming challenge. By explaining each step in this process, *The Breast Health Checklist* will reduce your anxiety, give you a greater sense of confidence, and allow you to be a proactive participant in your own healthcare.

The Breast Health Checklist is a practical resource for women who have breast symptoms, who need a breast biopsy, or who are diagnosed with breast cancer. In fact, the information in this book will be of value to any woman concerned about breast health, including women who want to reduce their risks through diet and lifestyle choices and stay healthy by performing self-exams. At the end of the book, special sections contain blank forms designed to create a permanent record of your mammograms, doctor contact information and visits, and other breast healthcare. The checklists in this book include important questions to ask your doctors that will allow you to become a proactive patient, involved in every step of your treatment and recovery.

You can keep this book at home to use as a reference source, and you can carry it with you to your appointments. Bring this book with you to routine mammograms to log the date of your exam and record the results in the appropriate section at the back of the book. The Breast Health Diary section will also be valuable for use in documenting biopsies or any treatments that might be needed. Recording all of this information in one place will transform this book into a handy resource for tracking all of your personal breast healthcare. In the event that you should need breast surgery, bring this book with you to the hospital or surgery center. When you register and fill out the required questionnaires, the information that you have entered into the medications and supplements lists, the doctor contact list, and the insurance information page will be very useful. If you choose to go for a second opinion, the Breast Health Diary will contain the most important information that you will want to bring to a new doctor. Checklists in this book will also help you to ask your doctor relevant questions in a variety of situations, such as receiving a diagnosis of dense breasts, DCIS, or breast cancer. If you are considering elective surgery, in order to make an educated decision, other checklists include specific questions to ask your doctor. There are lists of relevant questions specific to breast reconstruction, breast reduction, and breast enlargement.

The Breast Health Checklist will not only educate you about breast health; it will also empower you to take control of your own healthcare.

Rand J. Stack, MD
WESTMED Medical Group
Rye, New York

Understanding the Breast and Breast Health Awareness

BEFORE WE GET TO THE FIRST CHECKLIST, let's place in historical context the topic of breast health, as well as the development, structure, and function of the breast. Understanding the composition and function of the breasts will provide a foundation for information offered throughout this book on breast symptoms, risk factors, and breast health screening for the purpose of detecting breast cancer at the earliest stage.

Bringing Breast Health into the Open

Until the 1970s, breasts were not considered a polite topic of conversation, and women with concerns about the health of their breasts would hesitate to seek professional advice. The medical field was dominated by often-authoritarian male doctors, and many women dreaded the prospect of discussing intimate matters (including their breasts) with a physician. Tragically, some women with lumps in their breasts or bloody nipple discharge avoided doctors and essentially died of embarrassment.

Breasts indirectly became the topic of public discussion in the 1960s when the emerging women's movement orchestrated public "bra burnings." The book *Our Bodies, Ourselves*, first published in 1971, was written by feminists in response to their concerns that the healthcare system did not respect women or adequately address their health concerns. The authors also recognized that women at that time were not knowledgeable about their own bodies and women's unique health issues. Limited information about the breasts was scattered through that groundbreaking book. *Our Bodies, Ourselves* became widely read, and gave women permission to talk candidly about their bodies without embarrassment.

Betty Ford deserves enormous praise for her role in making breast health a subject of public discussion. Just weeks after becoming First Lady of the United States, on September 28, 1974, Betty Ford underwent a mastectomy for breast cancer. At a time when women usually kept this diagnosis secret, the First Lady announced her diagnosis and treatment to the American people. Just two weeks later, Margaretta "Happy" Rockefeller, the Second Lady, also had a mastectomy, and made her diagnosis public as well. Suddenly, breast cancer (and breast health in general) shifted from a hushed-up, private secret to an acceptable topic of public conversation. Important information about the signs of breast cancer was widely disseminated, and instructions for breast self-examination were published in popular women's magazines.

As a result of breast cancer activism, breast cancer reached the stature of a major public health issue in the 1990s and government funding for breast cancer research increased dramatically. The pink ribbon became a symbol of breast cancer awareness and was quickly ubiquitous. The importance of breast health to the American public was confirmed in 1992 when Congress passed the Mammography Quality Standards Act (MQSA). This legislation was created to ensure that all women would have access to high-quality mammography as an effective way to screen for breast cancer and to close facilities that performed subpar mammography.

Structure of the Breast

It may surprise you that the breast is a highly specialized variation of a sweat gland. The main structure of the breast is the mammary gland. In our mammal ancestors, the mammary gland evolved from a typical sweat gland that produced cooling perspiration into an organ for producing nutritious milk. Milk forms in the mammary gland and travels through a system of ducts that merge, forming larger and larger ducts as they travel toward the nipple. This pattern is like a landscape with streams joining to form rivers that come together as they travel toward the ocean. All the small milk ducts in the breast merge into between eight and fifteen major ducts, which each open separately on the nipple. Since these ducts each have a separate opening at the surface of the nipple, when milk is expressed from the breast it sprays in multiple streams, like water coming out of a showerhead, rather than in a single stream, like water coming out of a bathtub faucet. Tiny muscle fibers are arranged around the ducts. These fibers can contract to squeeze milk out of the ducts—and into the mouth of a hungry infant. The branches of the duct system end in lobules at the ends of each branch, like bunches of grapes at the ends of grape stems. Milk is produced in the lobules and travels down the ducts to the surface of the nipple. Breast tissue is very sensitive to hormones, which control the development of the breast and the production of milk.

The breast is composed primarily of three components: glandular tissue, fibrous tissue, and fatty tissue. The glandular tissue includes the lobules that secrete milk and the ducts that carry milk. The fibrous tissue includes structures called Cooper's ligaments, which support the lobules and ducts. Between the lobules are varying amounts of fatty tissue, which in some women may comprise a large proportion of the breast. The internal structure of the breast may be compared to the internal structure of a pomegranate. The white membranes that divide the pomegranate into segments are comparable to the Cooper's ligaments in the breast. The tightly packed seeds of the pomegranate are comparable to the many lobules that secrete milk, one at the beginning of each duct.

Every part of our body is composed of cells. The cells that line the lobules at the ends of the milk ducts are the location where most breast diseases occur. Like every part of the body, blood vessels travel through the breasts to provide the breast tissue with its essential blood supply. In tandem with the blood vessels, lymphatics branch through the breasts. This network of thin ducts helps clear the breasts of foreign materials, unwanted fluids, and germs. In all parts of the body, the lymphatics drain to lymph nodes that remove foreign materials and bacteria. After passing through the lymph nodes, the filtered lymphatic fluid travels through the lymphatics and empties into major veins. The lymphatics of the breast drain to several groups of lymph nodes, primarily those located in the armpit on the same side. Some lymphatic drainage from the breast may also go to lymph nodes located above the collarbone, or to internal mammary lymph nodes behind the breastbone. Cancer cells from a tumor within the breast may travel to any one (or more than one) of these lymph node groups.

The nipple is composed of skin and erectile tissue, which allows the nipple to stand erect when a woman is breastfeeding, cold, or sexually aroused. The skin surrounding the nipple, the areola, is pigmented pink or brown, depending on a woman's complexion. During the last trimester of pregnancy, the areola becomes larger and more deeply pigmented to make it more conspicuous, and therefore easier for a blurry-eyed newborn to find when nursing. It is normal for a number of small bumps to appear on each areola. These bumps are sebaceous glands, called the glands of Montgomery. Their function is to excrete oil that moisturizes and lubricates the nipple and areola. These bumps may become more pronounced during pregnancy. Oftentimes, a few hairs are present at the outer edge of the areola as well, which is absolutely normal.

Breastfeeding

Breasts exist for the purpose of feeding infants milk. The words *mama*, *mammal, mammary gland*, and *mammogram* all come from the Latin word for *breast: mamma*. This Latin word is believed to originate from the *mmm, mmm* sound of an infant suckling at the breast. There are many benefits of breastfeeding, both to the child and to the mother. Human milk is the healthiest food for a newborn infant. It contains precisely the right proportions of fat, protein, and other nutrients to provide the baby with optimal nutrition. Breast milk contains hundreds of nutrients that support a baby's health and growth. In addition to providing ideal nutrition, only breast milk contains antibodies that can transfer the mother's immunities to her infant and thus help the baby to fight infections. A baby cannot make antibodies to fight an infection until he has been exposed to the specific germ that causes the infection. Therefore, it is important for a woman to transfer antibodies to her baby through breast milk. This will protect the baby from germs that his mother has fought in the past. The World Health Organization recommends that every mother attempt to breastfeed her newborn, and that she should begin within thirty minutes of childbirth.

It is a good idea for nursing moms to take a vitamin D supplement, to ensure that the milk provides complete nutrition for the baby without depleting the mother's body of her own resources.

Breast Development

There are five basic stages of breast development in women:

- *Stage 1: Immature.* Prior to puberty (the physical changes of adolescence), only the nipple projects away from the chest wall.

- *Stage 2: Breast bud stage.* The nipple and breast project away from the chest wall as a small mound. The areola increases in diameter.

- *Stage 3: The breast and areola continue to grow larger.* The contour of the areola parallels the contour of the surrounding breast.

- *Stage 4: The areola projects forward from the contour of the breast*, as a second mound rising above the mound of the breast.

- *Stage 5: Mature stage.* The breast is fully developed, and the areola no longer projects beyond the breast contour.

Breast development begins when a buttonlike breast bud forms behind each nipple. This is one of the first changes of puberty. The breast bud develops into the mammary gland, giving the developing breast its shape. If a surgeon inexperienced with children were to mistake the breast bud for a mass and remove it, breast development would never occur on that side. On average, puberty occurs in African American females about one year earlier than in Caucasian American females. In recent decades, puberty has occurred in females at progressively younger and younger ages. According to the textbook *Gynecology: A Clinical Atlas*, the average age of puberty among girls has decreased from 17 years in 1830 to 12 years in 1980. Various explanations have been proposed for this trend, including improved nutrition, widespread obesity, and chemical contaminants in the environment. It is possible that this trend is the result of hormones given to dairy cows to increase milk production, which are secreted into cows' milk and consumed by young girls.

When breast development is complete, it is very common for one breast to be noticeably larger than the other. This is normal, and should not be cause for concern. Asymmetry of the breasts is not a risk factor for breast cancer. If there is a large difference in the sizes of your breasts, you may correct for this with special bras or, in extreme cases, with cosmetic surgery (see chapter 9). A rare congenital birth defect called Poland syndrome prevents one breast from ever developing. Babies born with this syndrome lack a pectoral muscle in the chest on the affected side and often have one or more missing arm bones on the same side of the body. During puberty, there is no breast bud, and consequently no breast development on the affected side.

Occasionally, a girl is born with an extra nipple. Extra "ectopic" nipples (or breast tissue) may develop anywhere along an imaginary "milk line" that arcs along the left or right half of the front of the torso from the armpit to the groin. A woman with ectopic breast tissue may find that, during pregnancy, the ectopic breast tissue enlarges simultaneously with her two breasts. A woman with an extra nipple may discover that it produces milk when she nurses her infant. Rarely, a woman may have three fully developed breasts. When this occurs, the third breast is always located along the left or right milk line. Historic documents from sixteenth-century England indicate that the second wife of King Henry VIII, Anne Boleyn, had three fully developed breasts. While this might certainly be factual, some historians believe that this allegation was part of a political smear campaign.

How to Use This Book

THIS BOOK IS NOT INTENDED AS A MEDICAL TEXTBOOK or even a complete encyclopedia of information on breast health for patients. Rather, this guide is a practical source of useful information for women with concerns about breast symptoms, including women who have been told that they need a breast biopsy and women diagnosed with breast cancer. The checklist format allows you to approach a wide range of breast health concerns in an organized and thorough fashion. For instance, if you have been told that you need a breast needle biopsy, the appropriate checklist will ensure that you arrive fully prepared for the procedure. The corresponding section on needle biopsy in chapter 5 will provide you with information to educate yourself about the procedure, reassure you, and dispel any unnecessary fears. If you have been newly diagnosed with breast cancer, the checklist on "Questions to Ask Your Doctor If You Are Diagnosed with Breast Cancer" in chapter 6 will enable you to ask relevant questions that will help keep you informed about the important details of your condition and help you anticipate the tests, treatments, and future outcomes that you are likely to face over the coming weeks and months.

Chapter Summaries

Chapter 1: Risk Factors
This chapter includes objective information about breast cancer risk and factors that increase a woman's risk of developing breast cancer. Here you'll find practical information that you can use to reduce your risk of developing breast cancer.

Checklist in this chapter:

☐ Actions That May Reduce Your Chance of Breast Cancer

Chapter 2: Breast Health Screening

In the event that you develop breast cancer, early detection can allow you to face treatment that is easier and less traumatic, compared to the treatment for advanced breast cancer. In fact, early detection can save your life. Following the steps in this chapter will maximize the likelihood that if a breast cancer arises it will be detected early. You'll also find easy instructions for breast self-examination, allowing you to literally place your breast health into your own hands.

Checklists in this chapter:

☐ Life-Preserving Screening Recommendations

☐ Signs of Breast Cancer When Examining Your Breasts

Chapter 3: Mammography & Breast Imaging

Whether you are about to go for your first mammogram or your thirtieth, this chapter will give you useful information to make the experience more comfortable, protect your modesty, and prepare you for additional procedures that might possibly be needed following the mammogram. You'll also find recommendations for scheduling and preparing for an MRI examination.

Checklists in this chapter:

☐ Preparing for Your Mammogram

☐ Questions to Ask Your Doctor If You Have Dense Breasts

☐ How to Prepare for a Breast MRI Examination

Chapter 4: Breast Symptoms

It is natural for patients with breast symptoms to experience anxiety. This chapter will help you to understand which symptoms are usually harmless and which symptoms require evaluation by a doctor.

Checklist in this chapter:

☐ Changes to Be Aware Of in Your Breasts

Chapter 5: Breast Biopsy

If you are scheduled to have a needle biopsy, this chapter will help you to anticipate what to expect. In addition, you'll find steps that may increase your comfort and reduce possible problems, such as bleeding, following the procedure.

Checklists in this chapter:

☐ If You Need a Breast Needle Biopsy

☐ Questions to Ask When a Needle Biopsy Is Scheduled

Chapter 6: Breast Cancer Facts

If you have been newly diagnosed with breast cancer, the information in this chapter will allow you to ask relevant questions that will keep you informed about the important details of your condition. This information will help you to anticipate the tests that you will face in the coming weeks and the treatments and future outcomes that you are likely to face over the coming months.

Checklists in this chapter:

☐ Questions to Ask Your Doctor If You Are Diagnosed with Breast Cancer

☐ Questions to Ask Your Doctor If You Are Diagnosed with DCIS

Chapter 7: Breast Cancer Surgery

If your doctor recommends a lumpectomy or a mastectomy, this chapter will allow you to prepare yourself for surgery and a possible overnight hospital stay, as well as minimize potential problems, such as arm swelling.

Checklists in this chapter:

☐ Questions to Ask Your Surgeon before Breast Cancer Surgery

☐ Lumpectomy Pre-Op Checklist

☐ Mastectomy Pre-Op Checklist

☐ Steps to Minimize Lymphedema (Arm Swelling) after Axillary Lymph Node Dissection Surgery

Chapter 8: Radiation & Medical Therapy

Radiation therapy and chemotherapy are unfamiliar experiences for most women diagnosed with breast cancer. This chapter provides information about chemotherapy regimens most often prescribed for breast cancer, including the advantages and disadvantages of different approaches. Other medications used for breast cancer are discussed as well.

Checklists in this chapter:

- ☐ What to Expect during Radiation Treatment
- ☐ Questions to Ask Your Radiation Oncologist before Radiation Therapy
- ☐ Things to Have with You during Radiation Therapy
- ☐ Questions to Ask If Your Doctor Prescribes Chemotherapy
- ☐ Preparing for Chemotherapy Treatments

Chapter 9: Reconstructive & Cosmetic Breast Surgery

Plastic surgeons are capable of bringing about remarkable transformations that can have an enormous positive impact on a woman's self-image. If you have had breast cancer and are planning to have reconstructive surgery, or if you are considering cosmetic breast surgery, this chapter includes valuable information as well as many important questions to ask your surgeon (and to ask yourself).

Checklists in this chapter:

- ☐ Questions to Ask before Breast Reconstruction Surgery
- ☐ Questions to Ask Yourself If You Are Considering Breast Enlargement Surgery
- ☐ Questions to Ask Yourself If You Are Considering Breast Reduction Surgery
- ☐ Questions to Ask If You Are Considering Breast Lift Surgery

At the end of this book, you will find a series of forms that will help you monitor your breast health. This section includes a chart for keeping track of your yearly mammograms and other breast imaging, as well as records of your prescription medications and insurance information that will be useful when you go to the doctor.

CHAPTER 1
Risk Factors

Risk Factors

Actions That May Reduce Your Risk of Breast Cancer

- ☐ Avoid hormone (estrogen) replacement therapy.
- ☐ Be a mother: Term pregnancies reduce risk.
- ☐ Breastfeed your infant.
- ☐ Maintain a lean body weight.
- ☐ Do not use tobacco products.
- ☐ Limit alcohol consumption.
- ☐ Avoid milk from cows treated with hormones.
- ☐ To the extent possible, avoid working night shifts.

CERTAIN CHARACTERISTICS OR BEHAVIORS ARE KNOWN TO BE ASSOCIATED with increased risk of developing breast cancer. Some of these risk factors, such as family history of breast cancer, are beyond a woman's control. Others, such as taking hormone replacement medications for menopausal symptoms, are avoidable. Although this chapter lists many breast cancer risk factors, it is important to keep in mind that 75–80 percent of women who develop breast cancer have *none* of the known risk factors. In other words, only 20–25 percent of women who are diagnosed with breast cancer fall into one or more of the categories identified as having higher risk than the general population. This means that no woman should feel that she can skip breast cancer screening because she is not at high risk. In fact, without question, the most important risk factor for breast cancer is being female. After all, 99 percent of breast cancer victims share this one risk factor.

Fortunately, there's no need to panic: with proper screening you can address any problems early, and certain steps can help you to manage or even reduce your risk. If you would like to estimate your own personal risk of developing breast cancer, you can use the online Breast Cancer Risk Assessment Tool developed by the National Cancer Institute (NCI). This tool, available at *www.cancer.gov/bcrisktool/*, calculates your risk of developing breast cancer at some time during your lifetime. If your estimated personal risk is 20 percent or greater, you might consider speaking to a breast surgeon or to an oncologist, a physician specializing in medical oncology, or the study of cancer, to discuss ways to manage your risk. You can find a breast surgeon by calling the office of your gynecologist or internist to ask for the names of breast surgeons to whom they refer patients. You can also ask nearby friends or relatives who have had breast surgery to recommend a breast surgeon. Alternatively, you can visit the website of your local hospital or women's health center and read the profiles of their providers.

High-risk patients may be monitored with vigorous screening or may take medications intended to prevent the development of breast cancer.

Family History

FAMILY HISTORY IS A VERY COMMON RISK FACTOR FOR breast cancer. If a woman's first-degree relative (mother, sister, or daughter) has had breast cancer, this confers a significantly elevated risk, particularly if the family member was diagnosed with breast cancer before menopause. Having a mother or sister with breast cancer triples a woman's risk. If both your mother and your sister (or two sisters) have had breast cancer, then your individual risk of developing breast cancer is six times as great as that of the general female population. Even having a second-degree relative with breast cancer increases your risk. If your aunt (whether maternal or paternal) or your grandmother (whether maternal or paternal) has had breast cancer, your risk is 50 percent greater than the general female population. Having two second-degree relatives with breast cancer doubles your risk. It is particularly important for women with a family history of breast cancer to have a mammogram every year, beginning at age forty (or even younger, if a mother or sister was diagnosed with breast cancer before age fifty).

I often read mammograms of women who were adopted as infants and therefore are unaware of their family medical history. Many of these women voice considerable anxiety over their situation. In fact, many of my adopted patients worry more about the possibility of developing breast cancer than do other patients with a known family history of breast cancer. I advise women who do not know their family history to assume that their lifetime risk of developing breast cancer is the same as the general population—12 percent—and I consistently recommend that they follow the "Life-Preserving Screening Recommendations" listed in chapter 2 of this book.

A PATIENT'S STORY

Family History and Breast Cancer

Jane was a vivacious thirty-four-year-old woman whose gynecologist found a lump in her breast during a routine exam, just before her final bridal gown fitting. Her physician sent her to me for an ultrasound examination of the breasts. The ultrasound images showed that the lump was solid, and I judged that it had a suspicious appearance, so I recommended a needle biopsy. The prospective bride had a needle biopsy later that day, which showed that the lump was breast cancer. The young woman put her wedding on hold to undergo a lumpectomy, radiation therapy, and chemotherapy. Her attentive fiancé stood by her through every step of her treatment and recovery. The would-be bride kept her sense of humor, maintained her positive attitude, and made a full recovery. The wedding was rescheduled to take place one year after the originally scheduled date. As the wedding date approached, the mother of the bride came to me for a routine mammogram. On the mammogram, I discovered suspicious calcifications, for which I recommended a needle biopsy. The biopsy proved that the mother, just like the daughter, had developed breast cancer. The mother of the bride vowed that she would not allow her own diagnosis to cast any shadow over her daughter's long-awaited wedding. She kept both the diagnosis and treatment secret from everyone, except her husband and her sister. She scheduled a lumpectomy to take place while her daughter was away on her honeymoon, and then quietly made daily trips to the hospital for radiation treatments. The bride did not discover what had happened to her mother until many months later. Now more than ten years have passed, and I continue to see the bride and her mother once a year, when they come for their annual mammograms. Both women are cancer-free, and they proudly bring me up-to-date on the accomplishments of the younger woman's growing children.

....

Genetic Risk Factors

THE RISK FACTOR THAT CONVEYS THE HIGHEST RISK of developing breast cancer (besides being female) is a BRCA gene mutation. The term *BRCA* stands for BReast CAncer, and to date, two different BRCA gene mutations have been identified. Families with BRCA gene mutations tend to be characterized by multiple women diagnosed with breast cancer before the age of forty, have a high incidence of cancer of the ovary, and often include men with breast cancer. Women who possess the BRCA-1 gene mutation have a 72 percent lifetime risk of developing breast cancer. Women with the BRCA-2 gene mutation have a 69 percent lifetime risk. This is in contrast to the general population of women, who have a 12 percent lifetime risk of developing breast cancer. Women with the BRCA-1 gene mutation also have a 44 percent risk of cancer of the ovary, and women with the BRCA-2 gene mutation have a 17 percent risk of cancer of the ovary. Keep in mind that BRCA gene mutations are uncommon, occurring in only 0.2–0.3 percent of the general population. Some ethnic groups have a higher incidence of these mutations, however. For instance, among women of Ashkenazi Jewish descent (Jewish populations that trace their heritage to Eastern Europe), the incidence of these mutations is ten times as great, at 2.5 percent.

The risk of developing breast cancer is so high for women with BRCA gene mutations that they are often screened more aggressively than the general population. For instance, BRCA-positive women are often screened with yearly MRI examinations of the breast, in addition to annual mammography and breast ultrasound. Some physicians order a breast ultrasound examination every six months for these high-risk women. The BRCA gene mutations do not occur only in women. Men who carry a BRCA gene mutation also are at risk of developing breast cancer. Although men are not normally screened for breast cancer, I recommend that men who are known carriers of a BRCA gene mutation be screened for breast cancer once a year with mammography.

Risk-Reducing Medications

The practice of screening women with a BRCA mutation with the combination of annual mammography, ultrasound, and MRI can detect breast cancer at the earliest stage that is currently possible. However, some patients who carry a BRCA mutation are not satisfied with early *detection* of breast cancer; they strive to *prevent* breast cancer from ever developing. Steps that have been taken to reduce the risk of breast cancer in these high-risk women include:

- Lowering estrogen levels by treatment with an anti-estrogen, such as tamoxifen or raloxifene (in postmenopausal women). These medications block estrogen receptors, and prevent estrogen from stimulating cancer cells.

- Lowering estrogen levels in postmenopausal women with an aromatase inhibitor, such as goserelin (Zoladex®). Fat cells are the major source of estrogen in postmenopausal women. Aromatase inhibitors prevent the formation of estrogen in fat cells by interfering with the enzyme aromatase.

- Removal of the ovaries.

The drugs currently approved for reducing the risk of breast cancer through lowering estrogen levels all have serious downsides that limit their use. Tamoxifen and raloxifene are associated with significant dangers arising from blood clots. Although aromatase inhibitors avoid this problem, these medications can cause serious bone loss. For these reasons, these medications are prescribed only to women who have a very high risk of breast cancer, including women with a BRCA gene mutation and women with a personal history of breast cancer. A more drastic treatment to reduce estrogen levels is removal of the ovaries. This is not universally recommended, but some women who have finished childbearing consider this option, since BRCA mutations are associated with an increased risk of ovarian cancer, and this step drastically reduces the risks of both breast cancer and ovarian cancer.

Prophylactic Mastectomy

A minority of women with a BRCA gene mutation elect to undergo prophylactic mastectomy of both breasts, to protect themselves from developing breast cancer in the future. *Bilateral prophylactic mastectomy* is the term used when both breasts are removed in a woman who has no history of cancer in either breast. This surgery is not performed as a treatment for cancer, since the patient has not been diagnosed with cancer. Women with the BRCA-1 mutation have an estimated 44–78 percent risk of being diagnosed with breast cancer by age seventy. Women with the BRCA-2 mutation have an estimated 31–56 percent risk of being diagnosed with breast cancer by age seventy. For women with BRCA gene mutations, it is estimated that bilateral prophylactic mastectomy reduces the risk of breast cancer by 47–90 percent.

The actress Angelina Jolie is an example of a BRCA carrier who did not have breast cancer but chose to have a double mastectomy to reduce her chance of developing cancer in the future. Women who choose to take this extreme step base their decision on the fact that they have a greater than 50 percent risk of developing breast cancer. It is important to understand that, even in the hands of an expert breast surgeon, following a mastectomy, 1 percent of the breast tissue will be left behind in the patient. Women with BRCA gene mutations who undergo prophylactic double mastectomy are not completely protected from developing breast cancer. However, by voluntarily having elective surgery, these high-risk women reduce their risk from ten times that of other women to the same risk of breast cancer as the general population of women.

Genetic Testing

Some readers may be wondering whether they should be tested for a BRCA gene mutation. It is important to clarify that BRCA testing is of great value to those women who are newly diagnosed with breast cancer, who have a strong family history consistent with a BRCA gene mutation, and who are facing a decision between mastectomy and breast-sparing cancer surgery (lumpectomy). Such a woman selects her treatment option based on the BRCA test result, choosing to have a lumpectomy if the test is negative and a mastectomy if the test is positive. Gene testing is *not* the right choice for every woman who is curious about whether she harbors a BRCA gene mutation but does not have breast cancer. Ashkenazi Jewish women are known to have a comparatively high incidence of BRCA mutations. However, even among this high-risk group, BRCA testing is not recommended for individuals without a diagnosis of breast cancer, unless there is a family history very suggestive of a BRCA mutation (e.g., multiple female relatives, or one male relative, with breast cancer).

Anyone considering BRCA testing should give very careful thought about whether or not testing is the right decision. First of all, unless a woman has multiple relatives diagnosed with breast cancer and/or ovarian cancer before the age of forty, she is unlikely to carry a mutation, and gene testing is not recommended. Secondly, a woman should not choose to be tested without thinking long and hard about how she would use the test information, in the event that the test turns out to be positive. If a woman is certain that a positive BRCA test will not prompt her to consider surgery (removal of the breasts and/or ovaries), medications that will make her infertile and cause symptoms of menopause, or yearly MRI exams, then the only result of a positive test would be increased anxiety. An example of a woman who would be an excellent candidate for BRCA testing would be a woman with a family history suggestive of BRCA who either has finished having children or is postmenopausal, and feels strongly that if she tests positive, she will choose to have prophylactic mastectomies and/or have her ovaries removed.

Even among women with a family history suggestive of a BRCA gene mutation, genetic testing is not always a good idea. For instance, an individual who suffers from anxiety should consider whether discovering that she has a gene mutation conferring a 65 percent lifetime risk of breast cancer might become an unnecessary source of additional angst.

Fortunately, there are laws in the United States that protect individuals from employment discrimination on the basis of genetic status, as well as laws that prevent insurance companies from limiting health insurance coverage on the basis of preexisting conditions. However, these laws do not apply to life insurance. Insurance companies are allowed to refuse to issue life insurance policies or to charge higher life insurance premiums to women who have tested positive for a BRCA gene mutation. A woman who anticipates that she might apply for life insurance in the future should investigate this issue and seek professional guidance before undergoing BRCA testing.

....

SHOULD I HAVE BRCA TESTING?

Do not get tested for a BRCA gene mutation unless you have a high likelihood of carrying the mutation, as shown by meeting two or more of the following criteria:

☐ You have been diagnosed with breast cancer before age forty.

☐ Many of your relatives have had breast cancer before age forty.

☐ Male relatives have had breast cancer.

☐ A close relative has tested positive for a BRCA gene mutation.

☐ You are of Ashkenazi Jewish descent.

Even if you meet these criteria, you should carefully consider what you would do differently should the test come back positive, compared to what you are currently doing.

....

Other Genetic Risks

In addition to the BRCA gene, dozens of other genes have been identified that are associated with increased risk of breast cancer. However, none of these genes impart a lifetime risk greater than 50 percent. I believe that additional undiscovered breast cancer genes exist that impart high risk of developing breast cancer equivalent to that of BRCA genes. This conviction results from my experience in medical practice seeing families with many women and often multiple men who develop breast cancer, yet test negative for currently known gene mutations. I have one patient whose family history is positive for mother, father, brother, uncle, two cousins, and two nieces with breast cancer. It is highly likely that this family harbors a breast cancer gene that has not yet been identified. One day this gene might be identified and named BRCA-3.

There are several rare genetic diseases that are associated with a high incidence of breast cancer. These include Cowden syndrome and Li-Fraumeni syndrome. These syndromes result in multiple distinctive medical problems, each with different key features. Interestingly, breast cancer is only a minor component of both syndromes. Both syndromes are rare, and Li-Fraumeni syndrome has been found only in a handful of families. Annual screening with breast MRI is officially recommended for three categories of patients with genetic risk of breast cancer: BRCA mutation carriers, Cowden syndrome patients, and individuals with Li-Fraumeni syndrome.

Age

Just as family history is a risk factor that you have no control over, age is a risk factor that you are unable to avoid. A woman's risk of developing breast cancer increases continuously as she ages. For this reason, I believe that screening recommendations that advise halting mammography at age seventy-four or at another age are ill conceived. You should never feel that you are too old to need a mammogram. I recommend that you continue having yearly mammograms until you reach the point that you are so debilitated that you would not choose to seek treatment for breast cancer, even if an early cancer were to be found.

Risk Factors You Can Control

WHILE YOU CAN'T HELP WHAT'S IN YOUR DNA, there are other breast cancer risk factors that are within your control.

Hormone Replacement Therapy and Contraceptives

For many decades, women were treated for hot flashes and other symptoms of menopause with hormone replacement therapy (HRT). It was eventually recognized that there is strong evidence that these hormones cause breast cancer, so they are now rarely prescribed. Many thousands of American women took these hormones for years. Clearly, this is a risk factor that is easy to avoid. If your physician prescribes hormone replacement therapy, think twice about following this recommendation. The temporary discomfort of hot flashes and other symptoms of menopause are generally not serious enough to justify the increased risk of breast cancer posed by hormone replacement therapy.

Oral contraceptive pills also contain hormones. There is very limited evidence for a link between use of oral contraceptives and breast cancer. However, doctors treating breast cancer patients generally recommend stopping use of oral contraceptives and switching to a different form of contraception, because estrogen is known to encourage the growth of many breast cancer cells. Taking this into account, I believe that it makes sense to avoid using oral contraceptives for years on end. In contrast to oral contraceptives, which include taking hormones twenty-one days out of every twenty-eight, transdermal contraceptives (birth control "patches" that adhere to the skin like self-adhesive bandages) and contraceptive implants that are inserted under the skin expose the body to continuous hormone influence. This represents continuous exposure of the body for long periods to hormones that are known to influence breast tissue. Although I am not aware of studies showing a link between these forms of contraception and breast cancer, you might consider avoiding these contraceptive methods as well.

Alcohol Consumption

One food product that has clearly been linked to breast cancer is alcohol. Women who consume three or more alcoholic drinks each week have a

15 percent higher incidence of breast cancer compared to nondrinkers. An international panel, the Collaborative Group on Hormonal Factors in Breast Cancer, published an article titled "Alcohol, Tobacco and Breast Cancer" in the *British Journal of Cancer* in 2002. The Collaborative Group reported that the incidence of breast cancer increases 7 percent with each additional daily alcoholic drink: 7 percent increased risk for one drink per day, 14 percent increased risk for two drinks per day, 21 percent increased risk for three drinks per day, and so forth. The explanation for increased incidence of breast cancer among women who drink may be an elevation of estrogen levels resulting from alcohol or may be related to DNA damage caused by alcohol. Limiting your consumption of alcohol is a very easy way for you to reduce your risk of developing breast cancer. Excessive consumption of alcohol is associated with many other diseases, including cirrhosis of the liver, pancreatitis, and increased incidence of many cancers, including cancer of the esophagus. Other consequences of excessive alcohol consumption include a higher rate of motor vehicle accidents and a negative impact on interpersonal relationships and employment.

Dietary Choices

When it comes to foods that can increase risk of breast cancer, the United States Food and Drug Administration (FDA) protects the American people from food products and medications that are harmful, including products that may cause cancer. However, small amounts of contaminants may find their way into some foods. For women who are concerned about breast cancer risk, it seems prudent to avoid foods that contain chemicals that have been shown to cause breast cancer. In light of the recognized link between hormone replacement therapy and the development of breast cancer, it seems wise to avoid food that contains excess hormones. It is a widespread practice on dairy farms for farmers to administer hormones to cows in order to increase milk production. These hormones are believed to find their way into the cows' milk, which is then consumed by humans. An easy way to keep these hormones from entering your body and the bodies of your family members is to drink only organic milk (or any milk from dairies that pledge never to give their cows hormones). You may also opt for almond milk or other nut milks that do not contain cows' milk.

Obesity

Another dietary factor associated with breast cancer is obesity. There is a higher incidence of breast cancer among obese women. This may be because fat cells secrete estrogen, and this estrogen may be the indirect cause of breast cancer in these patients. Therefore, maintaining a lean body weight is another way to reduce your risk of breast cancer. Admittedly, this is difficult advice to follow, especially for postmenopausal women who often struggle with their weight. However, like limiting one's alcohol intake, maintaining a lean body weight has multiple benefits in addition to reducing breast cancer risk. These benefits include lower blood pressure, decreased risk of diabetes, and fewer joint problems.

Smoking

There is evidence that long-term heavy smoking is associated with development of breast cancer. Additionally, there is a large amount of evidence that use of tobacco products can cause many potentially fatal health problems, including lung cancer, head and neck cancer, emphysema, and heart disease. I strongly recommend that you do not use tobacco products. If you are currently a smoker, please understand that this recommendation is not just another example of a doctor paying lip service to a tired old standard medical sermon. The cold, hard fact is that quitting smoking today is likely to do more good for your health than all of the other advice in this book! As discussed above, limiting alcohol consumption to one drink per day is another lifestyle choice that can reduce breast cancer risk and has many additional benefits.

Night Shifts

The International Agency for Research on Cancer (IARC) stated in 2007 that consistently working night shifts is "probably carcinogenic to humans." This conclusion was based on studies showing an increased incidence of breast cancer in women working night shifts. There is evidence that exposure to bright light during nighttime hours results in reduced blood levels of the hormone melatonin. It has been theorized that low levels of melatonin increase the risk of breast cancer by causing elevation of the blood level of estradiol (a hormone related to estrogen). Based on these studies, you might consider working daytime hours rather than night shifts, if you have a choice.

Breastfeeding

For women, breastfeeding is a painless lifestyle choice that has multiple benefits for both the mother and the infant (see page xiv). Among these benefits is lowering the mother's risk of developing breast cancer. While breastfeeding may not be an immediate option for every woman reading this book, if you are in the position to nurse, this lifestyle choice may help to reduce your breast cancer risk.

Four factors related to breast cancer risk may share a common pathway: late menopause, early onset of menstruation, breastfeeding, and childbearing. All four of these factors affect the number of menstrual cycles that a woman experiences during her reproductive years. Breast cancer incidence is increased among women who begin menstruating before the age of twelve as well as among women who experience menopause after the age of fifty-five. Breast cancer risk is decreased among women who bear children and among woman who nurse their infants. I suspect that the risk of breast cancer may be related to the number of menstrual cycles that a woman has during her reproductive years. Women who begin menstruating earlier or experience menopause later have a greater number of menstrual cycles. Women do not have menstrual cycles while they are pregnant, and women who are nursing often do not have regular menstrual cycles. Therefore, fewer menstrual cycles may be the common pathway to reducing the risk of breast cancer, potentially explaining why breastfeeding seems to reduce breast cancer risk.

Surgery

Surgery, the most effective measure to reduce risk of breast cancer, is so extreme that it is considered an option only for women with the highest risk. Surgery to reduce breast cancer risk may include removal of the breasts and/or removal of the ovaries. Some women who are diagnosed with cancer in one breast and receive a recommendation for a lumpectomy ask their surgeon to perform bilateral mastectomies instead. These women may decide to undergo surgery because they anticipate that they will be in constant fear of a second cancer, and they may wish to avoid the radiation therapy that accompanies a lumpectomy. It is important to realize that, even after the extreme measure of undergoing preventive surgery, a small percentage of patients may still develop breast cancer. This continued possibility of breast cancer is largely because some breast tissue always remains in the body following mastectomy, no matter how meticulous the surgical technique.

Surgery to reduce breast cancer risk is most often performed in women who are diagnosed with breast cancer and then discovered to carry a BRCA gene mutation (see page 5). If a woman diagnosed with breast cancer is found to carry a BRCA-1 gene mutation, her risk of developing cancer in the opposite breast during the next ten years is 48 percent. If a woman diagnosed with breast cancer is found to carry a BRCA-2 gene mutation, her risk of developing cancer in the opposite breast during the next ten years is 35 percent. By contrast, a BRCA gene mutation carrier who is treated for cancer in one breast and who has a mastectomy of the opposite breast is believed to have a risk of less than 1 percent of developing a future breast cancer.

Notes

_____

_____

_____

_____

_____

_____

_____

_____

_____

_____

_____

_____

_____

_____

_____

_____

_____

_____

_____

_____

_____

_____

_____

_____

_____

_____

_____

CHAPTER 2

Breast Health Screening

Breast Health Screening

Life-Preserving Screening Recommendations

☐ *Monthly:* Breast self-examination

☐ *Yearly:* Clinical examination of your breasts by your doctor or other healthcare provider

☐ *Yearly:* Mammography (starting at age forty)

☐ *Yearly:* Breast ultrasound: For those women whose breasts are extremely dense on mammography and for women with a personal history of breast cancer or a strong family history of breast cancer

☐ *Yearly:* MRI examination of the breasts: For those women who have tested positive for a BRCA gene mutation (or who have not been tested for the gene, but have a mother, sister, or daughter who is a carrier of a gene mutation)

CANCER SCREENING IS DONE TO CHECK PEOPLE WITH *no symptoms* for evidence of cancer. The goal of screening is to find cancer at the earliest stage, when it is most treatable. Early detection results in the best long-term health outcomes. Doctors routinely screen asymptomatic patients for colon, cervical, prostate, and breast cancer. Methods used to screen for breast cancer include mammography, clinical breast examination by a doctor or another healthcare provider, and breast self-examination.

Statistics from the American Cancer Society demonstrate that there was a 35 percent decrease in the number of breast cancer deaths in the United States between 1990 and 2014, coinciding with the introduction of widespread screening mammography. Although there has been well-publicized controversy regarding screening for breast cancer, the doctors on all sides of these arguments agree that women should have regular mammograms. The only thing these doctors argue about is how frequently screening mammograms should be done and at what ages screening should take place. A research paper, published in 2011 in the *American Journal of Roentgenology* by radiologists R. Edward Hendrick, MD, and Mark A. Helvie, MD, estimated the risk of death from breast cancer for the 20 million American women who were thirty to thirty-nine years old at the time they were writing. They concluded that screening these women with yearly mammograms starting at age forty would save 100,000 more lives, compared to screening these women with mammograms every two years beginning at age fifty. (For more scientific evidence that yearly mammography beginning at age forty saves women's lives, go to *https://www.sbi-online.org/endtheconfusion/Home.aspx.*)

The screening recommendations in this chapter are based on one single criterion: the steps that will bring about the greatest likelihood of discovering undiagnosed cancer in the breast, and therefore catching breast cancer when it is most curable and when it has not yet spread.

Breast Self-Examination

EVERY WOMAN SHOULD KNOW HOW TO PROPERLY EXAMINE her own breasts, and I recommend that every woman age thirty and older examine her breasts monthly. Some organizations have ended their former endorsement of breast self-examination based on the rationale that the number of harmless benign lumps found by women outnumbers the cancers that are discovered. Even though the yield may be low, the good that results from finding a cancer in one's own breast can be enormous. The best way that a woman can literally put her healthcare in her own hands is breast self-examination. Breast self-examination is the biggest bargain in breast health. It costs nothing, takes little time, requires no expensive equipment, and takes place in your own home. I see patients each year who have breast cancer that was discovered when the woman found a lump in her own breast.

By following these easy steps, you might save your life. One good way to remember to check your breasts every month is to examine them on the day that your period ends. This is a time in your cycle when the breasts are often the least tender. If you have gone through menopause or do not have regular periods, you might examine your breasts on the first day of each month.

Step 1: Visual Exam

Begin your self-examination by standing in front of a mirror and looking carefully at both uncovered breasts. First, stand with your hands on your hips, and look closely. Does one breast look different from the other? Next, stand with both arms raised over your head and look again. Look for any changes in your breasts compared to the past. Are both breasts the same size and shape? Do you see any dimpling or pulling of the skin? Does the skin look thickened, with prominent pores, like an orange peel? Is there any rash or redness? Has either nipple changed, or does the nipple look as if it is being pulled into your breast? Is there any crust, a sore, or a growth on the nipple or areola?

Step 2: Hands-on Exam

After examining your breasts with your eyes, you will examine them with your fingers. Use the pad of your fingers, the soft part that has the fingerprint. First, examine your left breast with your right hand. Either continue standing in front of a mirror or lie down on your back with a pillow behind your left shoulder and your left hand behind your head. Begin at the nipple, feeling for lumps in the breast. Slowly move your hand in clockwise circles around the breast, moving in bigger and bigger circles until you have covered the entire breast. Next, examine your right breast with your left hand. Stand in front of a mirror or lie down on your back with a pillow behind your right shoulder and your right hand behind your head. Begin at the nipple, and move your hand in counterclockwise circles around the breast. Some experts recommend examining each breast more than once, using light pressure to feel for abnormalities near the skin, and then repeating with firmer pressure to feel for lumps deeper down. If you have the time and patience to do this, it is a good idea. However, if the thought of going through this twice sounds like too much for you to do, it is better to examine each breast once than not to examine your breasts at all.

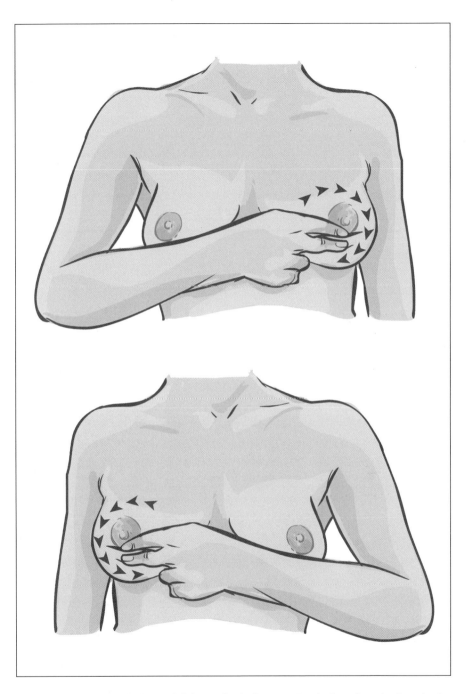

Use your right hand to check your left breast, beginning near the nipple and moving in a circular pattern outward over the entire breast. Then switch sides, using your left hand to check your right breast with the same circular pattern.

Step 3: Armpit Exam

The next step in breast self-examination is to feel for lumps in each armpit. This can be done while sitting or standing. With your arms at your sides and your elbows a few inches from your body, use your right hand to check your left armpit and your left hand to check your right armpit. If you notice any changes in your breasts or feel any lumps in your breasts or in your armpits, it is important to follow through by making an appointment with your doctor to show what you have found. Your doctor will examine you, and is likely to order a painless ultrasound test to check your breasts.

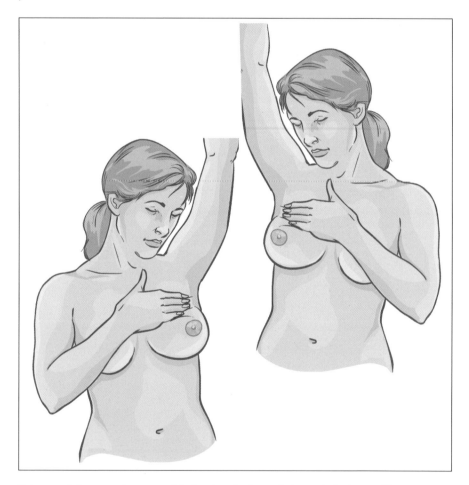

Raise your left arm, and use your right hand to check your left armpit for lumps. Then raise your right arm, and use your left hand to check your right armpit for lumps.

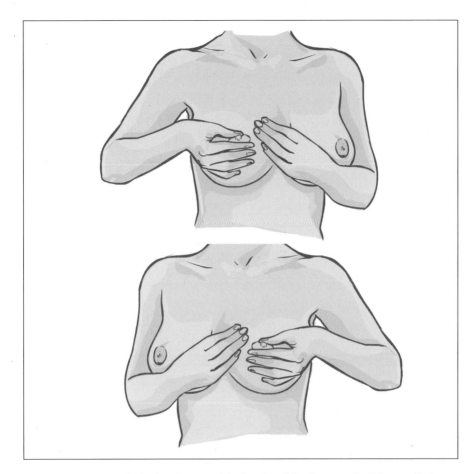

Gently squeeze your left nipple using your right thumb and forefinger to check for any discharge. Then switch sides to gently squeeze your right nipple using your left thumb and forefinger to check for any discharge.

Step 4: Check for Nipple Discharge

The final step in breast self-examination is to check for nipple discharge (droplets of liquid). Use your right thumb and forefinger to gently squeeze the left areola, including the nipple. Look for any discharge. If there is discharge, pay careful attention to the color. Nipple discharge can be straw-colored, bloody, green, or black (see page 45 for more on nipple discharge). After checking for nipple discharge on the left breast, repeat the process on the opposite side, using your left hand to gently squeeze the right areola, including the right nipple.

Signs of Breast Cancer
When Examining Your Breasts

- [ ] Lump
- [ ] Skin dimpling
- [ ] Bulge in contour of breast
- [ ] Skin thickened (like an orange peel)
- [ ] Prominent veins beneath the skin of one breast
- [ ] Nipple flattened or inverted (sunken below the surface of the breast)
- [ ] Nipple deviated or pointing away from the breast at an angle
- [ ] One nipple reddened or ulcerated
- [ ] Discharge from the nipple

Clinical Breast Examination

EXAMINATION OF AN ASYMPTOMATIC WOMAN'S BREASTS by a physician, nurse, or midwife is another important means of screening for breast cancer that has recently fallen out of favor with several respected organizations. Researchers have declared that clinical breast exams have a low yield of discovering undiagnosed cancers, and therefore they are not cost-effective. I am in favor of retaining routine clinical breast exams as part of every physical. Clinical breast examinations take very little time. In my opinion, a physician who performs a routine physical checkup or a routine gynecological exam is not doing a complete examination if he or she does not examine the breast for signs of breast cancer. Many cancers are discovered in this way. Since women under age forty do not normally have mammograms, clinical breast examination by healthcare providers is of particular importance for women in their thirties. In chapter 1, I recounted the story of Jane, a thirty-four-year-old bride-to-be whose gynecologist discovered a small lump in her breast during a routine checkup; that lump proved to be a cancer.

During the week that I wrote this paragraph, I cared for a sixty-year-old woman with advanced breast cancer who had been ignoring the growing lump in her breast, and carefully avoiding looking in the direction of the nipple that was becoming inverted. This intelligent, educated woman was in denial, and she did not seek medical attention for her worsening breast problem. But she did go to her gynecologist for her routine annual pap smear. The gynecologist wisely performed a routine clinical breast exam, discovering the cancer and setting the reluctant patient on the course to proper management of her condition.

Clinical breast examination requires no special equipment and can be performed by nurses, midwives, and physicians in many specialties, including family practice, internal medicine, gynecology, and endocrinology.

Screening Mammography

THE INTRODUCTION OF WIDESPREAD MAMMOGRAPHIC SCREENING for breast cancer is one of the great public health achievements of the twentieth century. For the fifty years leading up to the introduction of widespread mammography screening in the United States, the cancer death rate had been stable. Following the implementation of annual mammography screening for women age forty and older, there was a 35 percent drop in the breast cancer mortality rate in the United States, which has lasted for more than twenty years. Researchers Hendrick and Helvie estimated that women who have annual mammograms have a breast cancer death rate that is 40 percent lower than the breast cancer death rate of women who choose not to get mammograms.

Mammograms consistently detect DCIS (ductal carcinoma in situ), which is breast cancer at the earliest stage, stage 0. At this stage, all cancer cells are contained within the milk duct, and there has been no spread of cancer. By contrast, breast ultrasound, breast self-examination, and clinical breast examination (physical examination of the breast by a doctor or nurse) cannot usually detect breast cancer until it has progressed to an invasive stage and extended out of the duct into the surrounding tissue (see page 66). Although an MRI can sometimes detect breast cancer at the earliest stage, it cannot do so as consistently as mammography.

The Importance of Screening Mammography

Rosa, an eighty-one-year-old widow with arthritis, was scheduled for knee-replacement surgery. Her orthopedic surgeon instructed her to see her internist for medical clearance before the operation. The internist examined Rosa and judged that her physical condition was good enough to undergo surgery. Before officially clearing her, however, he ordered an EKG and standard blood tests. Rosa had not had a mammogram for four years, so the internist sent her to me for a mammogram. The mammogram revealed an unsuspected mass in the left breast. I introduced myself to Rosa and brought her into my office to discuss the mammogram. I explained that we had found an abnormality in her breast, and that she would need a needle biopsy. She listened carefully and told me, "First, I am having my knee surgery. I promise you that I will get this biopsy, but right now my knee is the most important thing." It took a great deal of convincing to persuade her that the breast mass was a more important health issue than the knee surgery. I alerted Rosa's internist that I believed the abnormality on the mammogram was breast cancer, and therefore the knee surgery needed to be postponed. I knew that six weeks of recovery from orthopedic surgery and physical therapy would not only interfere with scheduling breast surgery, it would also make five weeks of daily radiation therapy difficult. Despite her reservations about delaying her knee replacement, Rosa agreed to a needle biopsy of the breast mass, which was indeed cancer. She underwent a lumpectomy and radiation therapy. Rosa finally had her knee surgery three months later, after completing treatment for the breast cancer, and she was grateful to her doctors for insisting that she have a mammogram.

When to Schedule Your First Mammogram

Many large scientific studies performed in the United States and Europe, and published in respected medical journals, have demonstrated that the screening pattern that saves the most lives is yearly mammography, starting at age forty. For this reason I recommend that all women have a screening mammogram every year starting from the time they are forty years old.

In the case of a woman whose mother was diagnosed with breast cancer before the age of fifty, I recommend beginning yearly screening mammograms even earlier than age forty. If your mother had breast cancer before age fifty, I recommend that you start annual mammograms when you are ten years younger than the age at which your mother was diagnosed. For example, if your mother was diagnosed with breast cancer at age forty-four, then I recommend that you begin to have yearly mammograms at age thirty-four. The reasoning for this recommendation is that it is important to find a cancer at the smallest size and the earliest stage possible. Also, in my experience, women with a family history of breast cancer often develop the disease at a younger age than did their mothers.

Mammograms will be discussed in greater depth in the next chapter.

Breast Cancer Screening with MRI

BREAST MAGNETIC RESONANCE IMAGING (MRI) IS USED as a screening test only for women with very specific medical histories that place them at high risk of breast cancer. These uncommon risk factors are BRCA gene mutations, Cowden syndrome, Li-Fraumeni syndrome (see chapter 1), and a history of radiation therapy to the chest for Hodgkin's lymphoma between the ages of ten and thirty.

The next chapter will explore breast-screening examinations that require sophisticated equipment; this equipment generates images that are interpreted by physicians in one specialty—radiologists with additional qualifications in breast imaging.

Notes

_____

_____

_____

_____

_____

_____

_____

_____

_____

_____

_____

_____

_____

_____

_____

_____

_____

_____

_____

_____

_____

_____

_____

_____

_____

CHAPTER 3

Mammography & Breast Imaging

Mammography & Breast Imaging

Preparing for Your Mammogram

- ☐ Schedule your mammogram on days 7–10 of your menstrual cycle for maximum comfort.

- ☐ Bring a disk with your prior mammogram images, if this is your first time at the facility.

- ☐ Avoid wearing deodorant (perfume under your arms is OK—but it will sting if you shaved shortly before applying it).

- ☐ Wear a two-piece outfit, such as a blouse with slacks or a skirt. A dress or a jumpsuit will complicate uncovering your breasts for your exam.

- ☐ Wear sneakers, flat shoes, or low heels. You will be standing during your mammogram, and high heels may throw off your balance—especially if you are asked to lean forward or backward for better positioning.

- ☐ Take acetaminophen (Tylenol®) before your appointment if prior mammograms have been painful. (Avoid taking aspirin or ibuprofen, such as Advil® or Motrin®, for two weeks leading up to your mammogram in case you need a needle biopsy based on the mammogram. These medicines promote bleeding, and can remain in your blood for a week.)

THE FIELD OF MEDICAL IMAGING HAS DEVELOPED A VARIETY of technologies for detecting abnormalities of the breast. The most basic technique is mammography, which has benefited from exciting new developments in the twenty-first century. Other methods used for breast imaging include ultrasound, MRI (magnetic resonance imaging), and nuclear medicine imaging. These various imaging modalities each have different strengths. For instance, digital mammography is best at detecting DCIS (stage 0 breast cancer), ultrasound is best at differentiating cysts from solid masses, and MRI is best at evaluating breast implants for leakage.

What Is a Mammogram?

A MAMMOGRAM IS AN X-RAY EXAMINATION OF THE BREAST. An x-ray image of any body part is a picture of the shadow cast by x-rays when they are made to shine through that body part. Just as bright sunlight shining through a stained-glass window will cast a colorful shadow of the window's image on a church floor, the invisible x-ray beam will cast a detailed shadow of the interior of a body part, such as a hand or a breast, yielding an image that can be viewed on a computer monitor. The radiation dose of a mammogram is lower than the dose of any other medical x-ray examination. This dose is equivalent to the radiation exposure from cosmic rays that airline passengers get when flying from New York City to Los Angeles on a commercial airline flight.

Abnormalities, such as tumors in the breast, that block x-rays cast a shadow that is recognized by an experienced radiologist as suspicious. A radiologist is a medical doctor specializing in diagnostic imaging exams, including x-rays, ultrasound, and MRI. The breast is compressed between two plates for each mammogram image. Although the compression may be uncomfortable, it serves several important purposes:

1 Compression reduces the thickness of the breast, reducing the radiation dose needed to create a quality image.

2 Compression spreads out the breast tissue, reducing overlap of structures that might hide an abnormality.

3 Compression reduces involuntary motion of the breast that might result in a blurred exposure.

A standard mammogram includes two images of each breast: a side view and a view looking down at the breast from above. Under certain circumstances, additional views may be added to the screening mammogram. For instance, in rare situations a woman has breasts that are larger than the image receptor plate of the mammogram machine. In this case, it is necessary to take extra images in order to include parts of the breast that did not fit on the first four standardized images. In the case of a woman who has breast implants, additional images, called "implant displacement views," are obtained routinely, in order to evaluate a greater portion of those areas of the breast that are blocked by the breast implant on standard views.

Every mammography facility is required by the US government to notify patients of their mammography results within thirty days of a mammogram. This notification is usually in the form of a standardized "form letter" written in everyday language and mailed to the patient.

....

WHO READS YOUR MAMMOGRAM?

Mammograms are read by radiologists (medical doctors specializing in reading x-rays, ultrasound exams, CT scans, MRI, and other diagnostic imaging exams). Federal legislation passed in 1992, the Mammography Quality Standards Act (MQSA), requires that doctors reading mammograms have specialized training. The MQSA also requires interpreting physicians to read a minimum number of mammograms every year and receive at least fifteen hours in continuing medical education about breast imaging every three years.

....

Breast Density

"BREAST DENSITY" ON MAMMOGRAPHY REFERS TO how much of the breast is composed of glandular (dense) tissue and how much is composed of fatty tissue. There is no way for a medical professional to judge mammographic breast density by doing a clinical breast examination. For example, breasts that droop may be denser on mammography than breasts that are firmer to the touch. By definition, dense breasts are composed of more than 50 percent glandular tissue on mammogram images. Based on my personal experience reading thousands of mammograms every year for more than twenty years, I estimate that about half of women have dense breasts. The significance of dense breasts is that the dense glandular tissue may obscure a breast cancer on mammography. Some evidence confirms that women with dense breasts have a somewhat increased rate of breast cancer. At the time of this writing, thirty-two states have passed legislation requiring radiologists to inform women who have a mammogram if their breasts are dense. There is no consensus on whether women with dense breast tissue should do anything differently than women with breasts that are less dense. I recommend that women with breasts composed of greater than 75 percent glandular tissue undergo screening ultrasound of the breast in addition to annual mammography in order to look for abnormalities hidden by the dense tissue. I also believe that in women with breasts composed of greater than 50 percent glandular tissue, it is reasonable to add an annual breast ultrasound examination at the time of the annual mammogram if the woman also has a family history of a first-degree relative with breast cancer. First-degree relatives include a mother, a sister, and a daughter. I would also recommend both a mammogram and a breast ultrasound examination each year for a woman with dense breasts and a personal history of breast cancer.

There is a widespread belief among radiologists and gynecologists that young women tend to have mammographically dense breasts and older women tend to have breasts that are not dense on mammograms. Based on my experience, I believe that thin women generally have mammographically dense breasts and overweight women have breasts that are not dense. This is because thin women have predominantly glandular tissue in the breast and overweight women have predominantly fatty tissue in the breast. Standard tables of body mass index versus age show that women in the United States tend to gain weight as they age. I believe that those physicians who generalize that breasts become less dense as women age are attributing the change in breast density to aging, when it is actually the direct effect of weight gain (and only indirectly related to the aging process).

Questions to Ask Your Doctor
If You Have Dense Breasts

☐ Are my breasts moderately dense (50–75 percent glandular tissue)?

☐ Are my breasts extremely dense (75–100 percent glandular tissue)?

☐ Do you send your patients with dense breasts for additional imaging (ultrasound or MRI)?

☐ In the future, do you recommend that I have 3-D mammography, rather than conventional digital mammography?

Radiation Exposure and Mammography

A MAMMOGRAM IS AN IMAGE OF THE INSIDE OF the breast, taken with x-rays. Some women are concerned about the necessary exposure of the breasts to radiation during mammography. They worry that the radiation exposure of mammography may cause breast cancer. It is important to remember that the radiation dose during a mammogram is very low, even compared to other medical x-rays. To put this in perspective, we are all exposed to background radiation every day from cosmic rays that reach our bodies from outer space. This background radiation is greater at higher altitude. For example, a woman living in Colorado for six months is exposed to background radiation equivalent to the radiation exposure of a mammogram. In other words, if a woman in Colorado has a mammogram once a year, the background radiation exposure to her breasts between one mammogram and the next is double the radiation exposure of the mammogram itself.

The following evidence convinces me that mammography does not cause breast cancer: following the widespread introduction of screening mammography, a large number of women in America commenced yearly mammography, and statistics from the American Cancer Society show that the number of deaths from breast cancer dropped 35 percent. The overall decrease in breast cancer deaths vastly overwhelmed any possible tiny number of cancers resulting from mammograms. It would be a serious mistake to avoid mammograms out of fear that the radiation from the mammogram might induce a cancer in your breast. The only scientific evidence that has linked radiation to breast cancer is observation of an increase in breast cancer among Japanese women who were exposed to the nuclear blasts at Hiroshima and Nagasaki in 1945. However, these women were exposed to huge doses of radiation for a single instant. This is in no way similar to the minuscule radiation exposure that occurs once a year with a mammogram. Our bodies are designed to repair damage done by small injuries, such as low-dose radiation exposure, and this repair process can prevent the development of cancer. Furthermore, the breasts are thought to be most sensitive to radiation exposure when women are in their teens and twenties, ages at which mammography is not performed.

DIGITAL MAMMOGRAPHY VERSUS FILM MAMMOGRAPHY

The vast majority of mammography facilities in the United States perform digital mammography today. Digital mammography is superior to film mammography in multiple respects. Digital mammography uses a lower radiation dose, gives superior detail in dense breasts, and is clearly better at detecting microcalcifications, tiny deposits of calcium that appear as grouped dots on a mammogram. Since microcalcifications are the mammographic clue to detecting DCIS (stage 0 breast cancer), digital mammography is superior to film mammography at finding breast cancer at the very earliest stage. Finally, facilities that offer digital mammography are capable of utilizing computer-aided detection (CAD), which can help find more cancers. It is preferable to have mammograms performed at a digital facility than on an old mammogram unit that takes mammograms on films. Unless you live in a remote location where digital mammography is not available, I recommend having only digital mammograms (or 3-D mammograms, which are also digital) and avoiding facilities that perform film mammograms.

Computer-Aided Detection (CAD)

CAD IS A COMPUTER PROGRAM THAT ANALYZES THE DIGITAL mammogram images and points out findings on a mammogram that raise suspicions of breast cancer. CAD is possible only on digital mammography and 3-D mammography, and represents a significant advantage over film mammography. CAD is not meant to replace a human radiologist (a physician). The purpose of CAD is to help a radiologist focus on abnormalities, particularly if there are distractions in the room when the radiologist is working, and also to highlight findings that might be overlooked in dark areas or at the edges of the image. Typically, CAD will highlight multiple areas on a mammogram, and as part of the radiologist's examination of the images, he or she will study each of these areas, and generally disregard all (or most of them) as representing normal tissue. Currently available CAD systems typically use one symbol to point out suspicious microcalcifications and another symbol to point out possible masses.

I believe that it is an advantage to have CAD included with your mammography examination. Most insurance carriers agree that CAD adds value, and therefore they allow doctors to charge slightly more for reading mammograms when this adjunct is included.

Screening versus Diagnostic Mammograms

A MAMMOGRAM IS CONSIDERED A *SCREENING MAMMOGRAM* WHEN a woman with no breast symptoms is screened for breast cancer. The screening mammogram is usually performed when there is no radiologist on site, and screening mammograms are often read after the patient has left the facility. Radiologists typically interpret screening mammograms at a later time. I have worked in two practices that operated mobile mammography vans, in which technologists drove to office buildings and performed mammograms for the employees at the workplace. At the end of a day of performing mammograms at various office buildings, the technologists returned to the hospital with the mammogram images, which a radiologist would read at a later date. A screening mammogram usually includes four views (more views if the woman has breast implants or, rarely, if the breasts are larger than the image receptor of the mammogram machine).

By contrast, a *diagnostic mammogram* is performed when a woman has a breast symptom of concern, or when a woman has had an abnormality on a screening mammogram that requires further workup. A diagnostic mammogram is tailored to the particular woman's problem, and is normally performed under the direct supervision of a physician (that is, a radiologist).

Should your screening mammogram reveal an abnormality, your doctor may ask you to return for one or more of the following views:

- *Magnification views:* Used to evaluate calcifications to see if they are suspicious.

- *Spot compression views:* Used to evaluate suspected masses and confirm that they do not merely represent superimposed shadows of normal breast structures. When a woman is recalled to the mammography facility for spot compression views as part of the workup, her breasts are often examined with breast ultrasound on the same visit.

- *Tangential views:* Used to see if a calcification is in the skin, rather than in the breast. Calcifications in the skin cannot represent a breast cancer.

- *True lateral view:* Used to see if calcifications are liquid calcium ("milk of calcium") and therefore benign.

- *Cleavage view:* Includes the portion of both breasts close to the sternum (breastbone) to evaluate a suspected abnormality in this area that is not imaged on standard mammogram views.

3-D Mammography (Tomosynthesis)

THE MOST SIGNIFICANT TECHNICAL ADVANCE IN MAMMOGRAPHY during my twenty-plus years specializing in breast imaging is 3-D mammography. All previous mammography techniques resulted in images that superimpose all the structures in the breast one upon the other. As a result, normal structures could obscure a breast cancer by projecting over it in the image. This situation is a greater problem in dense breasts than in fatty breasts.

In contrast to this, 3-D mammography allows the radiologist to examine thin (1 mm thick) "slices" through the breast, one by one. Imagine a book with the words printed on pages made of transparent plastic sheets, instead of paper. Reading a digital mammogram (or a film mammogram) is equivalent to looking at thirty of these transparent printed pages stacked together, and trying to read the closed book without turning the pages. By contrast, reading a 3-D mammogram is like looking at each of the transparent pages, one at a time. Like digital mammography, 3-D mammography can detect microcalcifications, which is extremely important, because this capability allows radiologists to consistently detect DCIS (stage 0 breast cancer).

The unique strength of 3-D mammography is its ability to detect very small (stage 1) invasive cancers, which would otherwise be hidden in dense tissue. Since stage 1 cancers have a greater potential to prove fatal than do stage 0 cancers, this represents an important advance in mammography technology.

Breast Ultrasound

ULTRASOUND PLAYS AN IMPORTANT ROLE IN THE EVALUATION of the breasts. When a woman (or her physician) finds a breast lump, the most important step in evaluating the lump is ultrasound. This technique can reveal whether the lump is a harmless cyst (that is, water), a solid mass that requires a biopsy, or a "probably benign" finding that can be left alone for six months and then reevaluated with a repeat ultrasound examination. Ultrasound is the first test used to evaluate women under age thirty who present with breast pain, a lump, or a variety of breast symptoms. Ultrasound is the primary imaging modality for this age group because mammography is rarely done on these women. Ultrasound is also important for imaging women whose breasts are very dense on mammography, limiting the radiologist's ability to see abnormalities on mammograms. Another use of ultrasound is to examine women who have had a mastectomy, since mammograms are not used where there has been a mastectomy, even if there has been breast reconstruction surgery.

WHY CAN'T I JUST
HAVE AN ULTRASOUND AND
SKIP THE MAMMOGRAM?

Mammograms frequently detect breast cancer at the earliest stage, stage 0 (DCIS), when it is most treatable. Nobody dies of DCIS, because breast cancer never becomes fatal without first advancing beyond stage 0 to a more advanced stage. Therefore, mammograms are the only breast imaging modality that routinely detects breast cancer when it is most curable. If breast ultrasound had this same ability to detect breast cancer at the earliest stage, many women might prefer it to mammography, since it does not require compression of the breasts and does not involve radiation. However, breast cancer is usually not detectable on ultrasound until it becomes invasive and forms a mass (stage I, or an even higher stage). Since ultrasound typically detects breast cancer at a more advanced stage (invasive cancer) than is possible with mammography, ultrasound would not be an acceptable substitute for mammography as a screening exam.

....

Breast MRI

BREAST MRI (MAGNETIC RESONANCE IMAGING) IS THE MOST SENSITIVE technique for detecting breast cancer. However, MRI has some shortcomings as a screening test for breast cancer. MRI is expensive, requires an intravenous injection, and is not tolerated well by claustrophobic patients. However, the major shortcoming of MRI as a screening test for breast cancer is that there are many false positives (that is, false alarms). In other words, many benign (not cancerous) structures in the breast may look suspicious on MRI, requiring biopsies that subsequently turn out to be benign. For women at high risk, the likelihood of finding a true cancer on MRI is high, so the risk of false positives is less of a concern. Breast MRI is used as a screening test for women with the following uncommon high-risk factors: BRCA gene mutations, Cowden syndrome, Li-Fraumeni syndrome, or a history of radiation therapy to the chest for Hodgkin's lymphoma between the ages of ten and thirty.

Breast MRI has been used to evaluate women with newly diagnosed breast cancer. The purpose of performing MRI in these patients is to detect additional unsuspected cancerous breast tumors. This information can be important in choosing the best treatment for a woman with breast cancer. If a woman has multiple cancers in one breast, this information is important in planning her treatment, since a lumpectomy would remove only one cancer and leave other cancers within the breast. I have seen many cases where a woman had an MRI exam performed for a newly diagnosed cancer in one breast, and I found an unsuspected cancer in the opposite breast. In this situation, the woman was able to have lumpectomies in both breasts during the same operation and radiation therapy of both breasts simultaneously. I think this is a big benefit, since it spares her from having to go through the anxiety of being diagnosed with cancer in the second breast at a later date, undergoing and recuperating from surgery on two separate occasions, and going through five to seven weeks of radiation therapy five days a week more than once.

Some breast surgeons choose not to order an MRI exam to check women newly diagnosed with breast cancer for additional tumors. Their reasoning is that this practice has resulted in additional women choosing mastectomy, rather than lumpectomy. These surgeons seem to believe that their first goal is to save breasts by performing lumpectomies and avoiding mastectomies. I believe that we should not consider mastectomy to be our enemy; we should consider breast cancer to be our enemy, and recognize that, in select cases, mastectomy is the best treatment.

There are certain situations, other than screening for breast cancer, when MRI examination of the breast is valuable. For instance, breast MRI is the best method for evaluating breast implants for suspected rupture. Special MRI sequences (settings for the MRI scanner) are available that make it possible to highlight silicone and visualize whether it has leaked out of the breast implant into the adjacent breast tissue. To learn more about breast imaging modalities, go to *www.radiologyinfo.org*.

How to Prepare for
a Breast MRI Examination

☐ Make sure that your health insurance carrier precertifies the procedure prior to the date of the exam, and that the company pays the maximum benefit to which you are entitled.

☐ If you are claustrophobic, or feel that you would find it difficult to lie facedown with your arms above your head for 45 minutes, discuss the possibility of anti-anxiety medication with your physician (and arrange for a ride home so that you do not drive after being medicated).

☐ If you have any metallic devices implanted in your body, learn as much information as possible regarding what the device is, when it was implanted, and who manufactured it. Provide this information to the facility well in advance of the exam. Patients with cardiac pacemakers, implanted defibrillators, nerve stimulators, and cochlear implants are usually NOT candidates for MRI.

☐ You will have an intravenous line and an injection during the exam. If your veins are hard to find for blood tests, drink lots of fluids before the MRI exam so that your blood volume will go up. Check with your doctor if you believe that there is a reason that you should not drink to hydrate yourself at this time.

☐ Wear loose-fitting, comfortable clothing without metal parts (such as zippers, snaps, grommets, or buckles). You should wear a two-piece outfit, since you will remove your top and wear a gown for the exam.

☐ Avoid wearing any jewelry, except for gold rings, which are not attracted by the magnetic field. If you have a pierced nipple, leave the jewelry home.

☐ Do not wear anything metal in your hair: no hairpins, barrettes, or hair clips. The strong magnetic field in the scanner can rip these away, and they can become dangerous projectiles.

☐ Find out if the MRI facility has a sound system that allows patients to listen to music during the MRI scan. Ask the facility about bringing your own music to listen to during the MRI exam.

Notes

CHAPTER 4

Breast Symptoms

4 Breast Symptoms

Changes to Be Aware of in Your Breasts

- ☐ Nipple discharge
- ☐ Nipple inversion
- ☐ Heaviness
- ☐ Pain
- ☐ Itching or burning
- ☐ Sensitivity
- ☐ Skin retraction
- ☐ Lumps

BREAST SYMPTOMS OFTEN PROVOKE ANXIETY. Certain symptoms, such as a hard, painless lump in the breast, are reason to schedule an appointment with a physician, whereas others, such as diffuse tenderness of both breasts, rarely represent cause for concern. In particular, women with a family history of breast cancer tend to become concerned when a new breast symptom arises. The following descriptions should help you understand the significance of common breast symptoms.

Nipple Symptoms

MANY BREAST COMPLAINTS RELATE TO THE NIPPLE AND THE areola (the circle of pigmented skin surrounding the nipple). These include both subjective feelings, such as pain or itching, that are apparent only to you (referred to as "symptoms" by physicians) and objective changes that your doctor can see or palpate when she examines your breast (referred to as "signs" by physicians). Nipple pain, sensitivity, and itching are generally not suspicious symptoms. Nipple pain and sensitivity are generally related to hormones and commonly affect both nipples. Itching may be related to a more generalized skin condition. Nipple complaints that present as objective signs, such as nipple discharge, nipple inversion (retraction of the nipple below the level of the surrounding skin), and nipple discoloration, are of greater concern and may signify a serious problem.

Nipple Discharge

Two characteristics of nipple discharge indicate whether it is likely to be benign (harmless) or malignant (cancerous): the color of the discharge, and whether the discharge is from one nipple or from both. Discharge from both nipples is usually harmless. Discharge that is milky, yellow, or green is usually not important. Bloody discharge is far more often a sign of breast cancer. Bloody nipple discharge may be red, brown, or black. When a woman has bloody discharge from just one nipple, it is cause for serious concern, because it may indicate that a cancer is growing inside one of the milk ducts of that breast, and causing bleeding that travels down the duct to the nipple opening. Although bloody discharge is the most suspicious type of discharge, it may also result from a benign cause, particularly a mass called an intraductal papilloma, which grows within a milk duct. Although intraductal papillomas are benign, it is usually recommended that they be surgically removed when they are diagnosed by needle biopsy, because cancers can develop within them or alongside them. Milky discharge from both nipples is not considered a sign of breast cancer. Milky discharge is almost always the effect of elevated hormones, especially when it comes from both breasts. Women who have gone through menopause and later develop milky nipple discharge should be evaluated by a doctor, because it is possible that the cause of the discharge is an elevated level of the hormone prolactin in the bloodstream, possibly resulting from a tumor of either the adrenal gland or the pituitary gland.

Nipple Inversion

Nipple inversion (when the nipple retracts into the breast) is a very ominous symptom. There are some women who have had an inverted nipple since puberty, and this may be harmless. However, the new development of nipple inversion in an adult woman often indicates that a cancer is growing inside the breast, causing traction on breast structures such as Cooper's ligaments, or milk ducts, and pulling the nipple inward toward the mass. It is important to seek a physician's care without delay when nipple inversion develops. In fact, it is sensible to go directly to a breast surgeon, rather than to your primary care doctor, if you develop nipple inversion—assuming that your insurance carrier allows you to see a specialist without requiring a referral from a primary care doctor.

Nipple Skin Changes

Nipple changes that may seem innocent but are actually suspicious for cancer include the development of a sore, crust, or growth on the surface of the nipple or the areola. When these changes occur on one nipple, it is important to seek medical evaluation. This could represent Paget's disease of the breast, which results when breast cancer cells travel down the milk ducts to the skin of the nipple. Paget's disease can also present as redness, itchiness, or flaking of the nipple and areola. Keep in mind that redness, itching, or flaking of the nipple can also represent innocent dermatitis, particularly if these changes affect both nipples. However, it is not safe to assume that this is simply dermatitis, rather than breast cancer. The signs of Paget's disease may wax and wane over time. Therefore, it is possible for a woman to develop Paget's disease of the nipple, mistake it for dermatitis, treat it with cortisone cream, and erroneously believe that it is improving as a result of the topical medication when, in reality, she is only observing a temporary fluctuation in the manifestations of breast cancer.

Breast Issues

THERE ARE A VARIETY OF DETAILS ABOUT YOUR BREASTS that you may notice when doing a breast self-examination, when showering, or at any other time. One common observation is that the two breasts are slightly different in size or shape. This is comparable to having one foot slightly larger than the other, and therefore finding that whenever you try on a pair of shoes, one always fits better than its mate. Asymmetry of the breasts is extremely common, and unless it is a new development or it is accompanied by hardness of the breast or skin thickening, it is generally not cause for concern.

Breast Discomfort

A relatively common complaint among women with large breasts is a sensation of heaviness in the breasts. This is not a worrisome symptom, and it may be related to overall breast size or to generalized fluid retention. Wearing a bra with excellent support may alleviate this problem. Sometimes women with smaller breasts also complain of a sensation of heaviness, but this is usually not a cause for concern.

Other common symptoms that are almost always benign include breast pain and breast sensitivity. These symptoms are usually hormone related, especially when both breasts are involved. Among menstruating women, pain or sensitivity is most common in the premenstrual phase of the menstrual cycle. Hormone swings that occur around menopause may also result in breast pain or sensitivity. Sudden onset of severe pain in a band across one breast may represent shingles. This is a painful condition caused by the reactivation of the chicken pox virus that has been dormant inside a nerve for many years. The area of skin obstructing the branches of that nerve may develop extreme sensitivity and a rash. Tietze syndrome, inflammation of the front end of a rib where it meets cartilage, may mimic breast pain. Several ribs run beneath each breast, so this type of pain may be mistaken for breast pain if the involved rib is located behind the breast. Breast cancer is usually painless. It is very rare for breast cancer to present as breast pain. In my experience, in the rare instance that the first symptom of breast cancer is pain, it manifests as continuous deep pain concentrated in a single spot, like a toothache.

....

A PATIENT'S STORY

Caffeine and Breast Cysts

Maria was a sixty-three-year-old woman, sent to me for the first time after having had her previous mammograms and other breast imaging exams performed in another state. She came with a prescription for a routine mammogram, as well as a breast ultrasound examination. When her exams were done, I brought her into my office to give her the results. "Everything is fine. We just found a harmless cyst in your breast, and it can be left alone," I explained. Maria asked me, "How many cysts did you find?" After I confirmed that there was only one cyst, she told me that the reason she was curious was because "I used to feel like a farmer, growing cysts as my crop." Over a period of seventeen years, Maria had developed countless cysts in her breasts. During that period, she had gone through a total of nineteen needle aspiration procedures for these cysts. Triumphantly, Maria announced that four years ago, her doctor had suggested that she try giving up caffeine. Maria had previously been a devoted coffee drinker. After giving up coffee and all caffeine, she experienced a dramatic improvement in her breast symptoms. Maria was proud of her self-discipline, and delighted to learn that she now had only one cyst in her breast.

....

Cystic Breasts

Many women suffer with cystic breasts that become tender each month on the days before they menstruate. This can be the result of one or more cysts (fluid collections contained within a thin wall) that enlarge under the influence of the rising and falling hormone levels of the menstrual cycle. A woman may have dozens of cysts develop during her cycle. Less commonly, some women grow cysts the size of tennis balls. Cysts are completely harmless and do not develop into breast cancer. However, the presence of lumpiness in the breasts can be disturbing. Furthermore, it is more difficult to detect a lump that represents breast cancer in a breast that is full of cysts. This difficulty applies equally to physical examination of the breast and to mammography. In some, but not all women with cystic breasts, caffeine plays a role in the development of cysts. Some women with cystic breasts have found great relief from their monthly symptoms by eliminating caffeine from their diets. If you have cystic breasts and think that caffeine may be contributing to the problem, try a ten-week "caffeine-free challenge" (see checklist on next page). This involves eliminating all caffeine from your diet for ten weeks. Experience has shown that when caffeine is a contributing factor to cystic breasts, the symptoms will improve significantly following ten weeks without it. If there is no improvement after ten weeks, then you have established that caffeine was not part of the breast problem. Some women who have taken the caffeine-free challenge with no improvement in their breast symptoms have continued to avoid caffeine because they found that they were less anxious during the day and slept better at night. If you decide to try this challenge, please be aware that you must avoid *all* sources of caffeine, not just coffee, tea, and cola drinks. Chocolate contains caffeine, as do energy drinks and even decaffeinated coffee. Although you must eliminate all coffee, decaffeinated tea is allowed. Also, be cautious with soft drinks. Soft drinks other than cola may also contain caffeine, including a popular brand of citrus soft drink and some brands of root beer. It is important to read the product labels carefully.

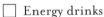

THE TEN-WEEK CAFFEINE-FREE CHALLENGE

For cystic breasts, try eliminating the following for ten weeks:

- ☐ Cola drinks
- ☐ Energy drinks
- ☐ All coffee (both regular and decaffeinated, also coffee candies and coffee ice cream)
- ☐ Tea (black tea, green tea, and white tea; however, decaffeinated tea and many herbal teas are allowed)
- ☐ Chocolate

If there is no improvement in the symptoms of cystic breasts after ten weeks, then caffeine is not a contributing factor and need no longer be avoided.

Fibrocystic Breasts

When the texture of a woman's breast is not uniform, but rather is lumpy, and she experiences breast tenderness that changes with the phases of her menstrual cycle, she is assigned the diagnosis of fibrocystic breasts (or fibrocystic mastopathy). This term implies that the breasts contain many cysts. However, this degree of diagnostic precision cannot be established by physical examination alone. The examining physician simply cannot know if palpable lumps correspond to cysts or solid masses or something else without the use of ultrasound or MRI. In fact, many women diagnosed with fibrocystic breasts have no abnormalities that can be found on mammograms or on breast ultrasound. In most cases, fibrocystic breasts are healthy and completely normal. Women with fibrocystic breasts often experience breast tenderness during the premenstrual phase of their cycles.

Skin Changes of the Breast (beyond the Nipple)

A variety of skin changes may affect the breast. These include rash, inflammation, skin thickening, and skin retraction. Women with sagging breasts who do not wear bras may have moisture trapped along the surface of the breast that lies continuously against the skin of the torso. In this warm, moist environment, bacteria and fungi may grow, causing a skin rash on the undersurface of the breast. This condition can be prevented by daily bathing, wearing a clean, comfortable bra with good support, and keeping the area beneath the breast dry.

Mastitis is an infection of the breast. This most commonly occurs in women who are nursing, and presents as reddened skin that is tender, thickened, and often warm to the touch. Mastitis is treated with antibiotics. Without treatment, mastitis may progress to formation of an abscess, a thick-walled collection of pus within the breast, which may require surgical drainage. One form of breast cancer—inflammatory carcinoma—causes reddening of the skin and may mimic mastitis. If a doctor treats you for mastitis and there is no significant improvement following a course of antibiotics, you should have a skin biopsy to check for inflammatory carcinoma of the breast.

Another skin change that may indicate breast cancer is skin retraction. Just as a malignant tumor of the breast may pull the nipple inward below the surface of the breast, breast cancer may retract the skin of the breast, causing it to indent toward the tumor, like a dimple. Development of this change is cause for serious concern. Equally ominous is the appearance of *peau d'orange* (French for "skin of an orange"). The skin of the breast becomes thick and firm, with the pores each forming a deep pit, like the indentations that pockmark the skin of an orange. This finding results from obstruction of the lymphatics that drain the breast. In patients with *peau d'orange*, the source of lymphatic obstruction is often breast cancer.

Breast Lumps

One of the most frightening breast changes is the discovery of a lump. Although the discovery of a lump causes many women to panic, most breast lumps are benign. Normal findings that may present as breast lumps include accessory breast tissue in the armpit and a prominent rib beneath the breast. The mammary gland is shaped like a teardrop, with a triangular extension—the tail of the breast—pointing toward the armpit. In some women, this may extend well into the armpit as accessory breast tissue, and may be palpable as fullness or as a lump. This tissue may become engorged with milk during pregnancy and lactation, causing the palpable lump to enlarge. Another normal finding that may be mistaken for a lump in the breast is a prominent rib located beneath the breast. This is most often discovered by a woman who has lost a considerable amount of weight. The breast consequently becomes smaller, and the rib is easier to feel.

> **Elongated lumps.** Elongated lumps in the breast that are much longer than wide are generally benign. A common elongated lump found on breast examinations is a curved ridge of firm tissue that follows the lower border of the breast where the breast meets the torso. I believe that this ridge corresponds to scar tissue, and that the formation of this ridge is the result of wearing underwire bras for a prolonged period. This is a harmless change that does not have any relationship to breast cancer. Another elongated lump that is often described as feeling like a cord under the skin of the breast is a clotted superficial vein, known to doctors as thrombophlebitis, or Mondor's syndrome. This is also harmless, and there is no danger of such a blood clot traveling to the lung or to any other part of the body.

Simple and complicated cysts. A round or egg-shaped lump within the breast may represent a cyst, a hematoma (blood collection), an abscess (pus collection), a benign solid tumor, or breast cancer. Doctors typically order an ultrasound examination of the breast to determine the nature of breast lumps. The most common breast lump, especially in younger women, is a simple cyst, which represents an encapsulated accumulation of water within the breast. Cysts are most often round, and they may reach a large size very quickly. Even though simple cysts are filled with water, they may feel hard when touched. Simple cysts have a characteristic appearance on ultrasound, so they can typically be identified as benign without the need for a biopsy. With the passing phases of the menstrual cycle, cysts may come and go, expand and contract. If a cyst is large and painful, it is possible for a doctor to insert a hypodermic needle into the cyst and draw out the liquid with a syringe, relieving the pain caused by the cyst and making the lump shrink away.

Not all cysts are simple. Complicated cysts (cysts with a thick wall, containing thick liquid or solid lumps) require more attention than simple cysts. They may be worked up with ultrasound-guided biopsy or managed with six-month follow-up ultrasound, depending on the individual appearance.

Hematomas and abscesses. Other fluid collections that may present as a breast lump are a hematoma (blood collection) or an abscess (pus collection). When a breast lump is a hematoma, it is usually easy to diagnose because there has been recent trauma to the breast and there is often a black-and-blue mark over the lump. A common cause of hematoma in the breast is a seat-belt injury following a motor vehicle accident. It may also be easy to diagnose a breast lump as representing an abscess when a woman has a fever and the skin over the lump is hot and red.

Fibroadenoma and lipoma. Another common benign lump in the breast is a fibroadenoma. These harmless lumps are usually oval- or egg-shaped and are most often found in young women.

Like fibroids in the uterus, fibroadenomas (also known as *fibroadenomata*) are composed largely of fibrous tissue. A small number of women form these benign tumors over and over again (a condition called fibroadenomatosis). If a needle biopsy proves that a breast lump is a fibroadenoma, then the lump has been proved to be harmless, and it can safely be left inside the breast. Fibroadenomas respond to hormone levels. They may grow during pregnancy, and they generally shrink after menopause.

In contrast to cysts and fibroadenomas, which tend to feel hard, lipomas are breast lumps that often feel soft or rubbery. Lipomas are benign fatty tumors that may occur anywhere in the body, particularly under the skin. Like cysts, lipomas can typically be recognized by their ultrasound appearance, therefore alleviating the need for a biopsy.

Breast Lumps during Pregnancy and Breastfeeding

Women often find lumps in their breasts when they are pregnant or during lactation (the period when they are producing milk after giving birth). These lumps may result from enlarging cysts or growing benign fibroadenomas, either of which may become larger under the influence of the hormones related to pregnancy and lactation. Additionally, milk ducts may become blocked, causing milk to back up and forming a sac filled with milk, called a galactocele. If mastitis (a breast infection) develops during nursing, this may progress to an abscess (a collection of pus) that can often be felt as a lump in the breast. Finally, benign glandular tissue in the breast may rapidly grow into a smooth lump under the influence of the hormones of pregnancy. This benign lump, called a lactating adenoma, can only be distinguished from a more serious abnormality by performing a biopsy.

Notes

CHAPTER 5

Breast Biopsy

Breast Biopsy

If You Need a Breast Needle Biopsy

☐ Avoid taking aspirin or ibuprofen (e.g., Advil or Motrin brand pain relievers) for two weeks preceding biopsy, unless instructed otherwise by your doctor.

☐ Bring a comfortable bra with no underwire to wear after your biopsy.

☐ Eat a light meal before the exam, unless you are instructed otherwise.

☐ Have acetaminophen (e.g., Tylenol brand pain reliever) available for pain.

☐ Apply cold to the biopsy site if you experience pain during the first few hours following the procedure.

☐ If you develop a black-and-blue area following the biopsy, apply a warm compress or heating pad, beginning the day after the surgery, to help the discoloration resolve more quickly.

APPROXIMATELY 2 PERCENT OF MAMMOGRAMS DETECT ABNORMALITIES that require a breast biopsy and, today, the vast majority of breast biopsies are performed as minimally invasive needle biopsies. The minimally invasive breast biopsy is truly a miracle of modern medicine. This minor "office procedure" does not require an operating room or general anesthesia (which always carries risks). As a consequence, the needle biopsy is safer and more economical than a surgical biopsy. The needle biopsy requires only a shallow injection of local anesthesia into the skin, like that injected in the mouth by dentists when filling cavities. No stitches are needed, so afterward, no stitches need to be removed. The procedure usually leaves only a tiny scar (about a quarter of an inch long), and often there is no scar at all. Finally, there is hardly any recuperation needed following a needle biopsy. The fact that the breast biopsy is so nontraumatic is significant, because the majority of breast biopsies—about 75 percent—turn out to be benign. Consequently, women who have minimally invasive breast biopsies with a benign result are able to avoid the operating room. Today, open surgery is essentially reserved for women with breast cancer (which was previously diagnosed by needle biopsy).

How Needle Biopsies Work

WHEN A NEEDLE BIOPSY OF THE BREAST IS PERFORMED, tiny bits of tissue are removed that resemble inch-long pieces of spaghetti. These biopsy specimens are made into microscope slides that are later examined under a microscope by a physician specializing in pathology. If the diagnosis is benign, then the major portion of the mass is left in the breast. Needle biopsy has been the standard of care for diagnosing breast lesions (abnormalities, such as lumps and calcifications) for decades. Millions of these minimally invasive procedures have been performed, with results approximately as accurate as more invasive surgical biopsies. During this period, there has been no evidence to suggest that needle biopsies spread breast cancer cells within the patient in any way. To guard against this unlikely consequence, when a patient undergoes lumpectomy surgery following a positive needle biopsy, the surgeon removes the nearby tissue that the biopsy needle previously passed through, eliminating concern that cancer cells were spread along the needle tract and might go on to grow there.

In the days before minimally invasive biopsy technology and needle localization techniques existed, a woman who had an abnormality discovered on a mammogram would often have open surgery that removed nearly a quarter of her breast, in order to be certain that the abnormal area was removed. The most unfortunate aspect of this outdated process was that, in the majority of these cases, this deforming surgery was needless, because the original mammographic abnormality represented harmless benign breast changes. Today, when a breast abnormality is found, a needle biopsy should be the first procedure in almost every case. If you have been told that you need to have a surgical biopsy in the operating room to determine whether or not you have breast cancer, you should ask your doctor tough questions about why he is suggesting open surgery, rather than starting with a needle biopsy. If you are not satisfied with the explanation that you are given, consider getting a second opinion from another breast surgeon. Your health insurance company will almost certainly cover the cost of a second opinion when surgery has been recommended.

Questions to Ask
When a Needle Biopsy Is Scheduled

- ☐ Will I need somebody to bring me home after the procedure?
- ☐ Will my activities be restricted following the needle biopsy? If so, for how long?
- ☐ When can I expect to learn the results of my biopsy? Who will contact me?
- ☐ How will I care for the biopsy site after the procedure?
- ☐ If the biopsy is positive, what will be the next step?
- ☐ Depending on whether you have an ultrasound-guided biopsy or a stereotactic (mammogram-guided) biopsy, you may be lying faceup or facedown during the biopsy. If you have spine problems or cannot lie in certain positions, ask your doctor about ways to accommodate your situation before the day of the procedure.

Types of Needle Biopsies

NEEDLE BIOPSIES CAN BE DIVIDED INTO TWO CATEGORIES: fine needle aspiration and core needle biopsy. The simplest kind of needle biopsy is called fine needle aspiration. The only equipment required is a needle and a syringe. The physician pulls back on the plunger of the syringe to create a vacuum and draw cells out of a lesion. This procedure retrieves only a small number of individual cells, which are smeared on a microscope slide and evaluated by a pathologist who is an expert in cytology (the microscopic examination of individual cells—distinct from cores of solid tissue). By contrast, core needle biopsy requires a special biopsy device that extracts cylinders of tissue from the breast. These cylinders contain intact breast tissue, rather than isolated cells, so studying them shows the actual tissue architecture of a portion of the lesion that has been biopsied. The tissue must be processed before it can be examined under the microscope. First it must be preserved in formalin (a solution of formaldehyde). Then it is embedded in paraffin wax. Next it is sliced into slivers thinner than sheets of paper. And finally it is stained to give the cell structures color. The resulting microscope slides can reveal minute details about the breast lesion to the pathologist.

There are two categories of biopsy devices used by physicians to perform core needle breast biopsies: spring-loaded devices and vacuum-assisted devices. The spring-loaded biopsy device takes tissue samples through spring action and makes a noise similar to an ordinary stapler each time the doctor takes a sample. With this type of device, the doctor typically takes approximately five tissue samples, and removes each sample from the biopsy device before taking the next sample. By contrast, the vacuum-assisted biopsy device usually includes an electric motor and a vacuum pump, which makes a noise like an electric sewing machine. This type of biopsy device allows the physician to take multiple tissue samples in rapid sequence without pausing in between each sample.

In order for a physician to successfully sample a breast lesion, she needs to know that the biopsy needle has entered the lesion. Unless the needle goes into the lesion, the significance of the abnormality cannot be diagnosed. In a case where the physician clearly feels a lump within the breast, it is possible to perform a needle biopsy without utilizing any diagnostic imaging technology. The physician first numbs the skin with local anesthetic, and then immobilizes the lesion with one hand on the patient's breast, trapping the lump between her thumb and forefinger. The other hand is used to carefully insert the biopsy device through the anesthetized skin, and into the lump.

More commonly, a breast lesion is identified on mammography, ultrasound, or MRI examination, and no lump can be felt in the breast. In these cases, an imaging-guided needle biopsy must be performed. The doctor may choose to do the biopsy using the imaging technology that revealed the lesion, or the doctor may choose the technology that is fastest.

There are some uncommon instances where a biopsy result is not breast cancer, but the lesion must still be surgically removed. One such situation is when the appearance of a lesion is highly suspicious for breast cancer on mammography, ultrasound, or MRI, but the biopsy result is read by the pathologist as either normal breast tissue or a benign abnormality that is not considered consistent with the appearance of the lesion on the images. In this case, the lesion is often surgically removed because of the possibility that the tissue that was sampled was not representative of the entire lesion, and therefore cancer cells may have been present in the lesion but not included in the biopsy sample.

A second uncommon situation sometimes occurs in which a lesion that is noncancerous must be removed following a needle biopsy. This is when the lesion is considered to be precancerous, or borderline malignant. The names of some lesions that are typically removed for this reason are *phyllodes tumor, radial scar, intraductal papilloma, atypical ductal hyperplasia* (ADH), and *lobular carcinoma in situ* (LCIS). These lesions are removed to make sure that there are no cancer cells within the immediate vicinity as well as to make sure that no precancerous cells are left behind that might potentially develop into a future cancer.

Ultrasound-Guided Biopsy

ULTRASOUND-GUIDED NEEDLE BIOPSY OF THE BREAST IS PERFORMED with the patient lying on her back on a table in the ultrasound room. This procedure is performed by a physician who may be a radiologist or a breast surgeon. An ultrasound technologist puts acoustic gel on the breast and scans the area of interest with an ultrasound probe. While the image of the mass is on the monitor, the physician numbs the skin with an injection of local anesthetic, and either the technologist or the physician holds the probe steady to provide a clear image of the biopsy as it takes place. The physician carefully inserts the needle through the anesthetized skin into the biopsy site. Then five or more tissue samples are removed with the needle. Afterward, an adhesive strip is placed over the skin to close the tiny wound where the needle entered.

Stereotactic Breast Biopsy

STEREOTACTIC BREAST BIOPSY IS PERFORMED with the patient lying on her stomach on a special x-ray table that has an opening in its center for the breast. The breast hangs down through this opening, and is compressed in a mammogram machine under the table. Stereo pairs of mammogram images are taken, with the two images in each pair taken at angles exactly 30 degrees apart from each other. A computer uses measurements from the paired images to calculate exactly where the target lesion is located (in three dimensions). These coordinates are transmitted to a mechanical needle holder, which guides the needle precisely to the location of the lesion within the breast. The physician typically uses the needle to take six to twelve tissue samples. Following the biopsy, a tiny metallic biopsy marker is placed through the needle and a stereo pair of images is taken to confirm that the marker was successfully deployed within the breast at the biopsy site.

MRI-Guided Biopsy

MRI-GUIDED BREAST BIOPSY IS PERFORMED with the patient lying on her stomach on the MRI table. Her chest is elevated above the tabletop on a raised frame, and the breast hangs through an opening in this frame. The breast is gently compressed (much less compression than for a mammogram) in a grid that is used by the radiologist to place the biopsy needle into the part of the breast corresponding to the abnormal area seen on MRI images. Performing a biopsy using this method is more time-consuming than ultrasound-guided biopsy or stereotactic biopsy. First, an MRI scan of the breast is performed. Next, gadolinium (a safe, intravenous contrast agent used for MRI exams) is injected into a vein in the patient's arm, and multiple postinjection image sequences are performed. The radiologist identifies the lesion on these images, and calculates its exact location. Next, the patient is slid out of the scanner, and the radiologist numbs her skin and marks the intended biopsy location with a hollow introducer that will be used to guide the biopsy needle. The patient is then slid back into the scanner, and another sequence of images is obtained. If the introducer is in the correct position, the patient is slid out of the scanner, and the needle biopsy is performed. Following the biopsy, the patient is slid back into the scanner, and a sequence of images is performed to confirm that the lesion was successfully biopsied. Finally, the patient is again slid out of the scanner, and a biopsy marker is placed through the introducer.

Biopsy Markers

THE FINAL STEP IN A CORE NEEDLE BIOPSY IS typically placement of a tiny metallic biopsy marker into the breast at the biopsy site. These markers are sometimes referred to as "clips," because the early models were designed to clip onto the tissue within the breast for the purpose of anchoring these markers in one place. The reason for using a biopsy marker today is to mark the biopsy site for future identification. After the biopsy samples are made into slides and evaluated under the microscope by a pathologist, it will be known whether or not the lesion in the breast represents a cancer. In the event that the biopsy proves positive for breast cancer, the patient usually undergoes a lumpectomy. A lumpectomy is surgical removal of the entire lesion, along with a small amount of surrounding normal breast tissue. In this case, the biopsy marker plays an important role, because it is used as a landmark to guide the surgeon to the exact spot of the biopsy. In this way, the lesion can be accurately located and removed. If the biopsy is negative for breast cancer, the biopsy marker is left in the breast and remains there for the patient's lifetime. When a marker is left in the breast, the patient cannot feel it, and it is not detectable by airport metal detectors. On future mammograms, the marker will be visible, documenting where the previous biopsy took place. Biopsy markers are manufactured in a variety of shapes. Doctors performing a breast biopsy generally endeavor to choose a biopsy marker of a shape that has not previously been used in the same breast.

CHAPTER 6

Breast Cancer Facts

6

Breast Cancer Facts

Questions to Ask Your Doctor If You Are Diagnosed with Breast Cancer

☐ Is the cancer ductal or lobular?

☐ Is the cancer in situ or invasive?

☐ What is the size of the tumor?

☐ What is the grade: low, intermediate, or high?

☐ What is the growth rate of the cancer: low, intermediate, or high?

☐ Does the tumor have receptors for estrogen (ER), progesterone (PR), or HER-2?

☐ What is the stage: stage 0 (in situ), stage 1, stage 2, stage 3, or stage 4?

☐ If you have had a lumpectomy or an excisional (surgical) biopsy, are the margins positive, negative, or close?

BREAST CANCER IS THE SECOND MOST COMMON CANCER of women in the United States (behind skin cancer), accounting for 29 percent of new cancers diagnosed in women. Most women dread the thought of being told, "*You have breast cancer.*" The first thing I hope to make clear is that a diagnosis of breast cancer is *not* a death sentence. In fact, 86 percent of women diagnosed with breast cancer will respond to treatment and will never die of the disease. With the discovery of aromatase inhibitors and HER-2-specific biologic therapy (see page 93), today there are better breast cancer treatment options than ever before. The majority of women diagnosed with breast cancer do *not* require mastectomy—and modern breast reconstruction techniques result in excellent cosmetic results for those patients who do undergo mastectomy. Finally, the introduction of sentinel lymph node biopsy (a technique that allows the doctor to sample just a few lymph nodes to establish whether the breast cancer has spread) has resulted in low rates of complications following breast cancer surgery. If you would like more information about breast cancer, go to the website of the National Comprehensive Cancer Network (NCCN), *https://www. nccn.org/patients/guidelines/cancers.aspx.*

Types of Breast Cancer

JUST AS THE TERM *CANCER* ENCOMPASSES MANY DISEASES, the term *breast cancer* encompasses two major types of cancer and several subtypes. Without counting carcinoma in situ (stage 0 cancer), the most common type of breast cancer is invasive ductal carcinoma. Ductal carcinoma and its subtypes account for about 80 percent of all breast cancers. Lobular carcinoma accounts for the majority of the remaining breast cancers. Rarely, other types of cancer may occur in the breast, including malignant phyllodes tumor, lymphoma, and metastases from cancers in other parts of the body.

Ductal Carcinoma

Ductal carcinoma arises from the cells lining the ducts through which milk travels from the glands where it is produced to the nipple, from which it exits the body. Ductal carcinoma typically forms a discrete solid growth in the breast that may show up on mammograms as a dense white shadow or on breast ultrasound as a solid mass that absorbs sound waves. When a ductal carcinoma becomes large, it will classically present as a hard, painless lump in the breast. A woman is typically diagnosed with invasive ductal carcinoma when it is seen on a routine mammogram as a mass (tumor), when she notices a lump in her breast, or when her doctor finds a lump during a routine breast exam. Less commonly, invasive ductal carcinoma of the breast is found when it causes skin retraction, bloody nipple discharge, or new development of nipple inversion (pulling in of the nipple below the level of the surrounding skin).

Several subtypes of ductal carcinoma have distinctive differences that are worth mentioning. Two subtypes of ductal carcinoma that are considered to be less aggressive than the typical variety are mucinous carcinoma (colloid carcinoma) and medullary carcinoma. Patients with these two types of ductal carcinoma can generally expect very good outcomes. Two other types of ductal carcinoma with distinctive features that are outwardly visible are inflammatory carcinoma and Paget's disease of the nipple. Because these forms of breast cancer both involve the skin, they change the outward appearance of the breast. Inflammatory carcinoma mimics a bacterial skin infection (cellulitis or mastitis). The skin becomes red, hot, and thickened. If your doctor treats you for these symptoms and they do not improve with a course of antibiotic therapy, you should be tested for breast cancer with a skin biopsy. Paget's disease presents as a sore, rash, or growth on one nipple or areola (the pigmented circle of skin surrounding the nipple). Symptoms of Paget's disease may also include itching of the nipple.

Lobular Carcinoma

Lobular carcinoma arises from the cells of the milk-producing glands that are present at the source of each milk duct. Lobular carcinoma can be very difficult to detect. It is harder to detect by clinical breast examination as well as by breast imaging, compared to ductal carcinoma. This is because ductal carcinoma typically forms a discrete mass that grows by expanding in every direction, whereas lobular carcinoma grows by extending tendril-like projections that burrow into the surrounding normal breast tissue. These thin, cancerous tendrils are difficult to detect, because they are only one cell wide, causing few detectable signs of their progress into surrounding tissue.

Breast Cancer Stages

ONCOLOGISTS, PHYSICIANS WHO SPECIALIZE IN CARING for cancer patients, use a formal staging system to classify each patient's cancer according to its type, size, severity, and location. This applies not only to breast cancer, but also to all cancers that arise in any organ, in any part of the body. A universal system of staging is published by the American Joint Committee on Cancer, and updated every few years.

If you are diagnosed with breast cancer, your doctor will determine the stage of your cancer to guide her in determining the appropriate treatment for you. This staging will also allow your doctor to follow your progress throughout your treatment. The earliest stage of cancer is stage 0 and the most advanced stage is stage 4. The stage of breast cancer with the best prognosis (outlook for future health) is stage 0 and the prognosis becomes progressively less favorable with each successive stage, with stage 4 having the least favorable prognosis. Your cancer will be classified as:

- *Stage 0:* Also known as carcinoma in situ (DCIS or LCIS), there is no evidence of spread of the disease to adjacent tissue.

- *Stage 1:* Limited to a small tumor (less than 2 cm) that may spread into adjacent breast tissue, but NOT to lymph nodes.

- *Stage 2:* Includes tumors up to 5 cm with possible spread to as many as three lymph nodes of the armpit (on the same side), as long as the lymph nodes remain freely movable, rather than firmly attached to adjacent structures.

- *Stage 3:* Locally advanced breast cancer, including tumors of any size. Stage 3 breast cancer may spread into the chest wall or through the skin, and may spread to as many as nine lymph nodes in the armpit on the same side, as well as lymph nodes around the collarbone or behind the ribs on the same side of the chest.

- *Stage 4:* This cancer is metastatic (that is, it has spread beyond the breast and armpit) and may include tumors of any size and involvement of any number of lymph nodes.

Carcinoma in Situ

IF YOU HAVE HAD A BREAST BIOPSY and your doctor has told you that the pathology (or cytology) result showed breast cancer, it is likely that you were given at least two major pieces of information about the cancer:

- Whether the diagnosis is invasive cancer or carcinoma in situ

- Whether the cell type is ductal carcinoma or lobular carcinoma

These distinctions will make a difference in what your treatment will be, and in what the outcome is likely to be in the future. Carcinoma in situ is considered stage 0 cancer. It is the earliest stage at which cancer cells can be distinguished from normal cells, and it is the stage of cancer with the best prognosis (long-term outcome). If you are diagnosed with carcinoma in situ of the breast, you should feel reassured that no one dies of carcinoma in situ. However, it is important for carcinoma in situ to be treated, because if it's left untreated, it may progress to invasive cancer. It can then metastasize to other parts of the body, and may eventually prove to be fatal.

....

SURGERY FOR DCIS SAVES LIVES, JUST AS AIRBAGS IN CARS SAVE LIVES

Some doctors inaccurately claim that stage 0 tumors, also known as DCIS, need not be removed from the body with a lumpectomy. The basis of this statement is a belief that some patients with DCIS might never have their tumors progress to invasive cancer. Doctors holding this belief proclaim that tens of thousands of women are therefore subjected to unnecessary breast cancer surgery each year. This half truth—that most surgery for DCIS is unnecessary—is equivalent to the statement that millions of consumers are paying unnecessarily for airbags in their cars, since only a tiny percentage of those airbags will ever be deployed. Just as we are not able to predict which new cars will be in collisions, we are not able to predict which stage 0 breast cancers will progress to invasive cancer and cause fatal metastatic disease. Therefore, surgical treatment is the standard of care for all patients diagnosed with stage 0 breast cancer.

....

As described above, the two major types of breast cancer are ductal carcinoma and lobular carcinoma. Both types begin their development at stage 0: ductal carcinoma in situ (DCIS) and lobular carcinoma in situ (LCIS). Physicians tend to treat DCIS more aggressively than LCIS. This is because DCIS is considered more likely to progress to more advanced stages than is LCIS. Some physicians treat LCIS as if it were a precancerous condition (rather than cancer) or a high-risk lesion that predicts an increased likelihood of a future cancer developing anywhere in either breast. Following a lumpectomy for DCIS, it is standard practice to perform radiation therapy; following a lumpectomy for LCIS, radiation therapy is usually not necessary.

Questions to Ask Your Doctor
If You Are Diagnosed with DCIS

- [ ] What is the grade: low, intermediate, or high? (The grade is the risk of the cancer advancing to invasive cancer if left untreated.)
- [ ] Was the tissue tested for receptors? Was it positive for estrogen? Progesterone? HER-2?
- [ ] If you have had an excisional (surgical) biopsy or a lumpectomy: Are the surgical margins clear?
- [ ] Does your doctor recommend radiation therapy for DCIS?
- [ ] Will you be receiving hormone therapy? If yes, when and for how long?
- [ ] Should you have genetic testing?

Metastasis

THE MAJORITY OF WOMEN DIAGNOSED WITH BREAST CANCER TODAY will not develop metastatic disease. An estimated 20–30 percent will have cancer spread to parts of the body away from the breast. Growing tumors may spread directly into adjacent structures, including ribs, muscles of the chest wall, and the skin of the breast. Cancer cells may also travel through the bloodstream or through the lymphatics to distant parts of the body, most commonly the bones, brain, lungs, or liver. If cancer has metastasized, it is typically treated with a systemic therapy, such as hormone therapy or chemotherapy, that will travel throughout the entire body, attacking cancer cells anywhere they may be, whether they have been detected by doctors or they are hidden and undiscovered.

Receptors

CELL RECEPTORS ARE A FEATURE ON THE SURFACE OF some breast cancer cells. These receptors act like switches that can turn cell functions on or off when they receive a specific signal. That signal arrives in the form of a specific molecule traveling through the bloodstream. The presence of cell receptors on breast cancer cells represents a unique opportunity for treating breast cancer, because very specific therapy can be used to target these receptors and deactivate the cells, causing them to stop flourishing. Therapy targeted to cell receptors is less toxic than chemotherapy and has fewer adverse side effects, making it a valuable breast cancer treatment. When pathologists examine breast tissue from a biopsy or lumpectomy and find cancer, they study the cancer cells to determine whether cell receptors are present.

The receptors most commonly identified on breast cancer cells are estrogen receptors and progesterone receptors. Estrogen and progesterone are hormones that play an important role in the menstrual cycle and breast development. Breast cancer cells that possess estrogen receptors and/or progesterone receptors will flourish in the presence of these hormones. Women whose cancers test positive for these receptors can be treated with medications that directly block these receptors. Alternatively, breast cancers that are hormone-receptor-positive can be treated by lowering the level of estrogen in the bloodstream, either through medication or (less commonly) through surgery.

HER-2 (human epidermal growth factor receptor 2) is another important receptor that may be present on breast cancer cells. This receptor is sometimes referred to as ERBB2. The importance of this receptor was first recognized in 1992. Breast cancer cells with extra HER-2 receptors on their surface exhibit amplification of the HER-2 gene, which makes breast cancers more aggressive and difficult to treat with conventional chemotherapy. Before the importance of this gene was recognized, patients with amplification of the HER-2 gene were not identified, and they had worse outcomes than other breast cancer patients. Now, targeted therapies have been developed that selectively attack cells positive for HER-2 receptors. These therapies are highly effective; as a result, patients positive for HER-2 now have a better prognosis, rather than a worse prognosis, compared to patients who are negative for all receptors (that is, triple negative). There are currently multiple laboratory tests available to check for HER-2 receptors. In the event that a test for this receptor is indeterminate, it is important that the tissue be checked a second time, using a different laboratory test.

....

A PATIENT'S STORY

Cancer Survivor with a Breast Lump

Heather, a fifty-seven-year-old breast cancer survivor, came to my office for her annual mammogram, as well as a breast ultrasound examination. She happily told the receptionist that this month marked a personal milestone of twenty cancer-free years following her lumpectomy. Heather confided to the staff that she planned to go out for ice cream, later in the day, to celebrate this occasion.

First, Heather had a mammogram, which was normal. On her ultrasound examination, I found a small mass behind her right nipple that was new compared to all her previous ultrasound exams. When I told Heather that I was recommending a breast biopsy, she was overcome with disappointment and fear. I reassured her that the majority of breast masses are benign, and I explained that, even though she had been diagnosed with breast cancer in the past, this mass was likely to be harmless. I made sure that Heather had a needle biopsy the next day. A few days later, the pathology report was ready and the mass proved to be benign. That evening Heather finally celebrated her twenty-year cancer-free anniversary—with ice cream.

....

Notes

CHAPTER 7

Breast Cancer Surgery

Breast Cancer Surgery

Questions to Ask Your Surgeon before Breast Cancer Surgery

☐ Which is the best operation for me: lumpectomy or mastectomy? Why?

☐ Will the choice of lumpectomy versus mastectomy make a difference in whether or not I also receive radiation therapy?

☐ Will I stay in the hospital overnight?

☐ What should I expect my recuperation to be like?

☐ Will I need to change dressings or care for my wound in any special way?

THE FIRST STEP IN THE TREATMENT OF BREAST CANCER is most often surgery. Cancer surgery (lumpectomy or mastectomy) removes the tumor from the body, or, in the case of carcinoma in situ, removes the cancer cells. Many breast cancer patients also receive additional treatment, such as chemotherapy or radiation therapy. Using surgery to reduce the amount of tumor in the breast makes chemotherapy and radiation therapy more effective.

Lumpectomy

THE MOST COMMON SURGICAL TREATMENT FOR BREAST CANCER IS lumpectomy. The term *lumpectomy* is misleading, because the word sounds like a description of the surgical removal of any lump from the breast. However, the term is only used to describe cancer surgery that removes a malignant (cancerous) lesion from the breast—even if there is no associated lump. The terms used for the surgical removal of a benign (not cancerous) lump from the breast are *excision* or *excisional biopsy*.

The term *lumpectomy* implies that a tumor can be easily shelled out of the breast. In reality, surgery for removing a cancer from the breast is more involved than opening a peanut shell and pulling out a nut. The edges of the lesion often fade into the surrounding normal tissue, making it difficult to tell exactly where the cancer ends. In fact, on a mammogram, a classic appearance of breast cancer is a sunburst pattern, with a central mass featuring rays radiating out from the cancer into the surrounding breast tissue. These extensions act like roots or tendrils, anchoring the tumor firmly in place. A longstanding principle of cancer surgery is that the surgeon cannot just remove the cancer, but must include an adequate margin of normal breast tissue all around the tumor. Some of the skin directly over the cancer is removed, along with breast tissue, during a lumpectomy. This skin typically includes the site of the needle biopsy that was previously performed, when the diagnosis of breast cancer was made. *Oncoplastic surgery* is a modern term used to describe cancer surgery that is modified specifically to obtain an improved cosmetic result. One example of oncoplastic surgery is use of the keyhole incision of breast reduction surgery to adjust the position of the nipple during breast-conserving cancer surgery.

Following every lumpectomy, a physician specializing in pathology examines the tissue that was removed from the breast to make sure that no cancer reached the outer edge of the surgical specimen. Sometimes a surgeon must bring a patient back to the operating room on a future date to take additional tissue to achieve clear margins and confirm that no cancer cells are left behind in the breast.

Lumpectomy is the standard surgery for breast cancer, but, in certain cases, this is not an option, and a mastectomy must be performed instead. Situations where a lumpectomy is *not* possible include:

- The cancer is too big to remove and yield a cosmetically acceptable result.

- The cancer involves more than one quadrant of the breast.

- The cancer involves the skin of the breast.

- The patient has had previous radiation therapy in the same breast.

- The patient is not capable of complying with five weeks of daily radiation therapy.

A lumpectomy is usually performed as outpatient (same-day) surgery. Before the patient goes to the operating room, she will typically undergo a procedure called needle localization. This most often takes place in the Radiology Department. A doctor (usually a radiologist) marks the location of the cancer cells in the breast to direct the surgeon to the exact spot. Taking this step enables the surgeon to safely remove the smallest amount of breast tissue possible. The radiologist uses either special mammogram equipment or an ultrasound scanner to find the lesion that will be removed in the lumpectomy. If a clip was previously placed in the breast to mark the location of a needle biopsy, the clip will serve as an important landmark during this procedure. During the needle localization, the radiologist first numbs the skin of the breast, and then inserts a needle containing a thin wire. After confirming that the needle is in the proper position, the needle is carefully removed, leaving only the thin wire extending out of the breast, like a cat's whisker.

Following the needle localization, the patient is brought to the operating room and an anesthesiologist administers an appropriate anesthetic to ensure that the patient will be comfortable during the surgery. The breast surgeon makes an incision in the breast and removes the cancer, along with a rim of surrounding normal tissue to be sure that no cancer is left behind in the breast. A small amount of skin is removed at the same time. The wound is closed with sutures, and the tissue that was removed is processed into slides that will be examined by a physician specializing in pathology. After a short stay of no more than a few hours in the recovery room, the patient is sent home with stitches at the surgical site, and a dressing over the wound.

Lumpectomy Pre-Op Checklist

- ☐ Arrange to have a family member or a friend drive you to and from the surgery venue.
- ☐ Bring your insurance card.
- ☐ Make a list of all your medications, and bring it with you (see page 160).
- ☐ Do not eat or drink anything after midnight the night before surgery, unless instructed otherwise by your surgeon.
- ☐ If you take prescription medications each morning, ask your surgeon if each of these should be taken on the day of surgery.
- ☐ Alert your surgeon if you take a blood thinner or low-dose aspirin so that proper adjustments to your medications can be made in advance of your surgery date to prevent bleeding problems.
- ☐ Buy a soft, snug sports bra with the closure in front to sleep in following the surgery.
- ☐ Do not take aspirin or ibuprofen for two weeks before surgery, unless told otherwise by your surgeon.

Mastectomy

MASTECTOMY IS THE SURGICAL REMOVAL OF THE BREAST as a treatment for breast cancer. Long ago, mastectomy was the only surgery performed for breast cancer. Today, the majority of women diagnosed with breast cancer do not need a mastectomy and their treatment is lumpectomy instead. This smaller operation spares the breast, removing only the cancer and a surrounding rim of normal tissue. However, some women choose to have a mastectomy. Why? Because it gives them the peace of mind that the procedure minimizes the possibility of future cancer in the same breast, or to avoid the need for radiation therapy. The commonly performed mastectomy today includes removal of the mammary gland, the nipple, and much of the skin of the breast. Patients undergoing a mastectomy generally spend one night in the hospital following the surgery.

The majority of women who undergo a mastectomy choose to have breast reconstruction surgery to replicate the appearance of a breast. This can be done immediately, during the same operation as the mastectomy, or it can be done at a later date. In some cases it is possible to perform a skin-sparing mastectomy, which simplifies breast reconstruction. Some surgeons even offer select patients a nipple-sparing mastectomy, which involves removal of only the mammary gland. This can result in an excellent cosmetic outcome, with the natural nipple remaining in place. (See pages 79 and 80 for more about skin-sparing and nipple-sparing mastectomies.) Breast reconstruction surgery is optional, not a medical necessity, but health insurance carriers generally do cover it. Some women refuse breast reconstruction, and choose to be flat-chested on one side following their mastectomy. Since the chest muscles are spared during present-day mastectomies, the chest of a woman who refuses reconstruction surgery will resemble a prepuberty chest on the affected side (with the exceptions of a surgical scar and the absent nipple).

Mastectomy Pre-Op Checklist

☐ Arrange to have a family member or a friend drive you to and from the surgery venue.

☐ Make a list of all of your medications, and bring it with you (see page 160).

☐ Do not eat or drink anything after midnight the night before surgery, unless instructed otherwise by your surgeon.

☐ If you take prescription medications each morning, ask your surgeon if each of these should be taken (or not) on the day of surgery.

☐ Alert your surgeon if you take a blood thinner so that proper adjustments to your medications can be made in advance of your surgery date to prevent bleeding problems.

- [ ] Do not take aspirin or ibuprofen for two weeks before surgery, unless told otherwise by your surgeon.

- [ ] Bring your insurance card and a photo ID.

- [ ] Pack an overnight bag and expect to spend the night in a hospital bed.

- [ ] Bring all your medications to take during your hospitalization, and let your surgeon know that you have them with you.

- [ ] Bring your own sleepwear, robe, and slippers (you will not like the versions that the hospital provides), as well as a favorite pillow.

- [ ] Bring reading material and/or an electronic device and charger to pass the time during your hospital stay.

- [ ] If you are staying in the hospital overnight, I recommend Elizabeth Bailey's book *The Patient's Checklist: 10 Simple Hospital Checklists to Keep You Safe, Sane & Organized*. The book has excellent advice on how to prepare for your hospitalization, suggests items to bring with you, and includes helpful forms to complete throughout your stay to prevent medical errors and to keep track of important steps in your care.

Skin-Sparing Mastectomy

SKIN-SPARING MASTECTOMY IS A CANCER OPERATION TO REMOVE the breast tissue while preserving as much skin as possible, including the inframammary fold (the line at the bottom margin of the breast where the breast joins the torso). Skin that typically is removed during this procedure is the nipple and areola, as well as the biopsy site. These tissues are not spared, because they are considered to be at the highest risk for recurrence of breast cancer. Scientific studies have shown that the overall risk of breast cancer recurrence in patients who undergo this operation is nearly the same as the risk for patients who undergo a conventional present-day mastectomy. Like all mastectomy patients, women who undergo skin-sparing mastectomy do not continue to have mammography on the mastectomy side in the future.

Skin-sparing mastectomy is usually combined with immediate breast reconstruction. In fact, breast reconstruction surgery is made easier by preserving as much skin as possible. Patients who have reconstruction with implants require neither additional surgery for placement of tissue expanders, nor weeks of saline injections to gradually expand the implants to the ultimate size for surgical replacement with silicone implants.

Skin-sparing mastectomy is not an option for patients with inflammatory carcinoma of the breast, as their skin and skin lymphatics are known to harbor breast cancer cells. This operation is usually not offered as an option to women who smoke, because the effect of smoking on small blood vessels can result in skin breakdown following the surgery. This can be a problem in diabetic patients as well, because diabetes also affects small blood vessels.

Nipple- and Areola-Sparing Mastectomy

NIPPLE- AND AREOLA-SPARING MASTECTOMY IS A VARIATION on skin-sparing mastectomy that preserves the nipple and the areola, in addition to most of the skin of the breast. Preserving the nipple and areola can have a tremendous positive impact on a woman's body image following breast cancer surgery. However, because there is an increased risk of breast cancer recurrence (estimates range from 6 percent to 58 percent) when the nipple is preserved, surgery that spares the nipple and areola is not commonly done. One technique used to minimize the risk of recurrence in the nipple is to carefully surgically remove the central tissue directly behind the nipple during the operation. A disadvantage of this technique is the likelihood that the nipple will lose sensation and erectile function.

Axillary Lymph Node Surgery

AN IMPORTANT COMPONENT OF BREAST CANCER SURGERY is management of the lymph nodes in the armpit (axilla) on the side of the surgery. These lymph nodes are of tremendous importance, because the first place that breast cancer spreads is typically to the lymph nodes in the nearby armpit. For this reason, examining the lymph nodes of the armpit has traditionally been an essential step in establishing whether or not cancer has spread beyond the breast. If metastases are not found in the lymph nodes of the armpit, it is concluded that breast cancer has not metastasized (that is, spread) beyond the breast. On the other hand, if breast cancer cells are found in the axilla, this shows that the cancer has spread beyond the breast, and additional tests are needed to determine how widely the breast cancer has spread. Such tests enable doctors to determine the stage of the breast cancer.

Sentinel Lymph Node Biopsy

The field of breast surgery was revolutionized in 1994, when the first scientific paper was published describing sentinel lymph node biopsy for patients with breast cancer. Until that time, axillary lymph node dissection (see page 82), a wider operation to remove all the lymph nodes from the armpit, was used to determine whether breast cancer had spread to the lymph nodes. Sentinel lymph node biopsy quickly became the standard procedure for staging the lymph nodes in the armpits of women with breast cancer. Sentinel lymph node biopsy allows the surgeon to establish whether cancer has spread from the breast to lymph nodes in the armpit by removing only one to three lymph nodes. This technique drastically reduced the extent of surgery performed in the armpits of women undergoing surgery for breast cancer, and has decreased the number of women with the long-term complication of lymphedema (permanently swollen arm).

The procedure for sentinel lymph node biopsy starts approximately thirty minutes before the patient goes to the operating room, with the injection of a tiny quantity of liquid into the breast. This injection may include a small quantity of short-lived radioactive tracer, blue dye, or both. The injected material travels through the lymphatics of the breast to the armpit, and is collected by the lymph nodes. At the time of breast surgery, when the patient is anesthetized in the operating room, the surgeon is able to identify the sentinel node. This is the first lymph node (or nodes) to collect the injected material. This is done by visually observing blue dye in a lymph node or by detecting radioactivity in a lymph node with a small handheld radiation detector. The surgeon removes the lymph nodes, and is careful to avoid disturbing the nerves and blood vessels that travel through the armpit.

Axillary Lymph Node Dissection

The goal of axillary lymph node dissection is to remove all the lymph nodes from the armpit, regardless of whether or not they appear outwardly abnormal. Axillary lymph node dissection is not considered adequate unless at least ten lymph nodes are removed; in practice, surgeons remove an average of fifteen lymph nodes. This procedure is usually performed on patients who have had a positive sentinel lymph node biopsy showing breast cancer in a lymph node. In other cases, this procedure is performed on patients who have an enlarged hard lymph node in the armpit that has signs of cancer, but has not been biopsied. Finally, in the uncommon cases where a sentinel lymph node biopsy was attempted, but did not identify a sentinel node, axillary lymph node dissection is performed as a staging procedure to determine whether or not the breast cancer patient has metastatic disease.

Many important structures travel through the armpit, including the major blood vessels of the arm, the major nerves of the arm, and the lymphatics that drain excess fluid from the tissues of the arm. Performing extensive lymph node surgery in the armpit may result in damage to these structures. The most common complication of axillary lymph node dissection is seroma, a collection of blood plasma under the skin of the armpit that can temporarily interfere with motion of the arm. A less common but more significant complication of axillary lymph node dissection is interference with the lymphatic drainage of the involved arm, causing lymphedema. Lymphedema is swelling of the arm on the side of the surgery. This swelling may involve the entire hand and arm and can last a lifetime. Published scientific papers estimate the frequency of this complication to vary widely from as low as 6 percent to as high as 70 percent, depending on the exact surgery and the health of the patients studied.

This arm swelling is very difficult to treat, and may develop immediately after surgery, or may be delayed and develop years later. Uncommon complications include nerve injury, which can result in numbness of the upper arm.

Steps to Minimize Lymphedema (Arm Swelling) after Axillary Lymph Node Dissection Surgery

- ☐ Avoid having blood taken from the arm on the involved side.
- ☐ Try not to have intravenous lines placed in the hand or arm on the involved side.
- ☐ Avoid having blood pressure taken on the involved side.
- ☐ Do not use hot tubs or saunas. The high temperature can aggravate lymphedema.
- ☐ Wear work gloves when gardening or doing other activities that involve a risk of injuring the skin of the hand and introducing infection.

Notes

CHAPTER 8

Radiation & Medical Therapy

Radiation & Medical Therapy

What to Expect during Radiation Treatment

- [ ] Consultation with radiation oncologist
- [ ] CT scan performed for planning angle and dose of radiation therapy beam
- [ ] Tiny tattoo marks in the skin
- [ ] Five to six weeks of treatments, five days a week
- [ ] Fatigue following treatment
- [ ] Possible temporary skin reddening

THE PRIMARY TREATMENT FOR BREAST CANCER IS SURGERY to remove the known tumor from the body. Additional therapies are available to destroy breast cancer cells that may remain in the body after the tumor is removed. These therapies include radiation therapy, chemotherapy, and hormone therapy. In the case of lumpectomy, the entire breast is often irradiated to destroy any unsuspected cancer cells present in the breast following the surgery. In some cases, cancer cells are known to be present in metastases that have been found with a PET scan, a CT scan, or another test. Chemotherapy can treat metastases anywhere in the body, whether they have been identified or are too small to detect. For more detailed information about radiation therapy or chemotherapy for breast cancer, go to the website of the National Comprehensive Cancer Network (NCCN), *https://www.nccn.org/patients/guidelines/cancers.aspx*.

Radiation Therapy

Questions to Ask Your Radiation Oncologist before Radiation Therapy

☐ What is the purpose of radiation therapy in my case?
To shrink a tumor before surgery? To destroy a tumor?
To kill possible undetected cancer cells?

☐ How many sessions of radiation will I have?
Over how many weeks?

☐ Will I have radiation five days a week?

☐ Will there be a boost (see page 89) to the surgical site?

☐ What side effects can I expect?

RADIATION HAS BEEN USED AS A TREATMENT FOR CANCER since shortly after the discovery of x-rays in 1896. Radiation kills cancer cells by breaking the DNA strands necessary for the cells to multiply. Cancer cells are more sensitive to radiation than normal cells, because cancer cells divide much more rapidly and are not able to keep up with repairing DNA breaks. Radiation therapy is typically used to treat women who have recently undergone a lumpectomy for breast cancer. When the standard treatment shifted from removing the breast (mastectomy) to preserving the breast (lumpectomy), a cornerstone of treatment was the use of whole breast radiation to kill any cancer cells that might have been left behind when the tumor was removed. In one estimate, breast cancer treatment accounts for 20–25 percent of radiation therapy treatments in the United States. Besides treating patients following lumpectomy, radiation therapy may be used to treat patients with breast cancer recurrence at the surgical site or to treat metastatic cancer elsewhere in the body. In certain situations, such as patients whose breast cancer has invaded the chest wall, radiation therapy may be used to treat the tumor following mastectomy.

If your doctor believes that you will benefit from radiation therapy, the first step is a consultation with a radiation oncologist, a physician specializing in radiation therapy. The radiation oncologist will review your medical records and pathology report and he will examine you. The radiation oncologist will decide the form of radiation treatment that is best for you and will prescribe a course of radiation therapy. The radiation most often administered is whole breast radiation, with an external beam of radiation precisely aimed at the breast. Partial breast radiation therapy may also be administered with external beam radiation directed to the lumpectomy site, but today this is less commonly done. An alternative to external beam radiation is partial breast irradiation administered from within the breast, either in the operating room during the lumpectomy procedure or afterward, by intermittently placing a radioactive source inside a tube implanted temporarily within the breast. This tube is removed after the course of radiation treatment is completed.

Things to Have with You during Radiation Therapy

- [ ] Your own music
- [ ] Noise-canceling headphones to reduce outside sound when listening to your music
- [ ] Your own pajamas, nightgown, or robe to wear (instead of the standard gown)
- [ ] Eye mask if you are claustrophobic (be aware that the machine will pass in front of you, close to your body)

External Beam Radiation

The most common form of radiation therapy for breast cancer is external beam radiation. A linear accelerator generates a stream of electrons and converts these into a thin beam of radiation. The radiation oncologist plans the dose and angle of the radiation beams for the optimal treatment of the breast. During treatment, a computer aims the beam at the target area from many angles, while rapidly moving shutters of a precision device called a multileaf collimator that continuously adjusts to block radiation from going outside the planned treatment area.

Treatment planning involves multiple steps. Four or more tiny dots will be tattooed onto your skin for use as landmarks to ensure that your positioning is identical for every session of radiation treatment. This guarantees that the prescribed dose will be administered. These marks will also serve as a permanent record of the site of your radiation treatment, in the event that you ever need radiation again in the future. Treatment planning begins with a CT scan of your chest. This scan generates data that will be used by sophisticated computer processing to generate cross-sectional and three-dimensional computer simulations of your breast and the surrounding structures. The radiation oncologist will plan precise radiation beams that will approach the target area from multiple angles and deliver the ideal dose to the target area while simultaneously minimizing the amount of radiation exposure to nearby normal structures, particularly the lungs and the heart. Special care is taken to eliminate any unnecessary exposure to the heart when the nearby left breast is being irradiated. The state of the art in radiation planning today is use of a CT scanner. Any facility performing external beam radiation therapy today without using this technology is not providing the best care.

Electron Beam Boost

The radiation oncologist may prescribe a boost to one or two treatment areas. This is an extra session of radiation therapy performed by direct use of the raw electron stream that is generated by the linear accelerator, without first converting it into a radiation beam. Electrons have only a fraction of the penetration power of the radiation beam generated by a linear accelerator, with the consequence that they affect only superficial tissues, with little radiation reaching the underlying structures. For this reason, an electron beam boost is ideal for treating a surgical scar to reduce the risk that cancer cells remaining from the time of surgery will grow in the skin scar.

Implanted Radiation Source (Brachytherapy)

Brachytherapy is the term used for radiation therapy performed by placing a radioactive substance inside the body to bring the source of radiation as close to the target area as possible, ideally within the tumor, or within the surgical cavity from which the tumor was removed. The radiation source chosen for this form of therapy is a radioactive isotope that produces radioactivity that is capable of traveling only a very short distance in the body. This minimizes the irradiation of nearby normal structures, such as the heart and the lungs. Partial breast irradiation is administered after placing one or more catheters into the breast. These tubes remain in the body throughout the radiation therapy treatment, and are removed following the treatment. One technique involves inserting between ten and twenty tubes into the breast for up to one week. During this period, the patient returns for multiple treatment sessions, when radioactive material is temporarily introduced into the tubes and then removed. An alternate technique involves placing a single balloon catheter in the lumpectomy cavity at the time of the lumpectomy surgery, and inflating the balloon within the surgical cavity. Radioactive liquid is injected into the balloon once daily during radiation therapy treatments, and then replaced with nonradioactive liquid before the patient leaves the facility. After five days of treatment, the catheter is deflated and removed.

Intraoperative Radiation

Intraoperative radiotherapy is radiation aimed directly into the surgical cavity during the lumpectomy operation. A major advantage of intraoperative radiotherapy, compared to other types of radiation therapy for breast cancer, is that it takes place in a single session—as opposed, for example, to the twenty-five times patients receiving external beam radiation therapy are required to return for treatments. For immobile patients who cannot easily be transported to daily treatments, the availability of intraoperative radiotherapy can make lumpectomy an option for women whose only choice would otherwise be mastectomy. Besides requiring only a single treatment, intraoperative radiotherapy has other advantages. Because it is aimed directly at the tumor bed during surgery, with the covering skin and normal tissues moved away by retractors to either side, the radiation is administered directly where it is needed. For the same reason, nearby tissues can be blocked from the radiation. An electron stream or a radiation beam with low penetrating power is used so that deeper structures receive a minimal radiation dose.

Medical Therapy for Breast Cancer

MEDICAL THERAPY FOR BREAST CANCER INCLUDES THE USE of pills or intravenous injections to kill cancer cells anywhere in the body, or to create an environment that will prevent breast cancer from recurring in the future. These therapies are prescribed and administered by oncologists. Medical therapies include hormone therapy, biologic therapy, and chemotherapy.

Questions to Ask If Your Doctor Prescribes Chemotherapy

☐ What is the goal of giving me chemotherapy? To prepare me for surgery? To eliminate any hidden cancer cells? To treat metastases? To protect me from recurrence?

☐ Can alternative medications be administered instead? What are the advantages and disadvantages of each option?

☐ How many sessions will I have? Over how long a period?

☐ Which chemotherapy agents will I be receiving?

☐ Will the chemotherapy drugs go directly into my vein, or will I have an injection port implanted under my skin for the intravenous needle to enter?

☐ What side effects should I expect? Will I lose my hair?

☐ Is there anything I can do to lessen the likelihood of side effects or decrease their severity?

☐ Will I be receiving hormone therapy? If so, when and for how long?

Hormone Therapy

Hormone therapy is a targeted therapy that selectively acts on breast cancer cells without having an effect on most of the cells in the body. This contrasts with chemotherapy, which is toxic to a large proportion of the cells in the body, with widespread undesirable side effects. Unfortunately, hormone therapy is not an option for all patients, only for those women with breast cancers who have hormone receptors on the breast cancer cells (see page 70). These receptors may be for the hormone estrogen, the hormone progesterone, or both. Some endocrine therapy treatments act by lowering the level of circulating estrogen in the body. This minimizes the influence of a hormone that can stimulate the growth of estrogen receptor–positive breast cancer cells. Other endocrine therapy techniques act by administering a medication that selectively binds to the hormone receptors on cancer cells, preventing them from being stimulated by estrogen.

In pre-menopausal women, the main source of estrogen in the body is the ovaries. Endocrine therapy in pre-menopausal women with breast cancer is focused on temporarily suppressing the production of estrogen by the ovaries or permanently preventing the ovaries from producing estrogen, either by removing the ovaries with laparoscopic surgery or by use of a medication that permanently ends ovarian hormone production, or blocking the activity of estrogen by blocking the receptor. The most commonly prescribed hormone therapy for pre-menopausal women with breast cancer is tamoxifen. Wide experience has shown that continuing tamoxifen therapy for five years following breast cancer treatment is effective in reducing recurrences in pre-menopausal women with hormone receptor–positive breast cancer. Published research suggests that extending this period to ten years is beneficial, but this benefit must be weighed against certain risks associated with tamoxifen therapy, including an increased incidence of blood clots. Pre-menopausal women treated with tamoxifen will experience symptoms of menopause, including hot flashes.

In postmenopausal women, the main source of estrogen in the body is fat tissue. Within fat cells, the enzyme aromatase generates estrogen. Hormone therapy in postmenopausal women is based on the use of aromatase inhibitors to prevent fat cells from producing estrogen. Research has shown that five years of therapy with an aromatase inhibitor is slightly superior to tamoxifen in reducing the risk of recurrence in postmenopausal women with hormone receptor–positive breast cancer. Five years of an aromatase inhibitor following five years of tamoxifen has been shown to have a marked effect in reducing breast cancer recurrences. One disadvantage of aromatase inhibitor therapy is increased incidence of osteoporosis and fractures. New drugs that affect the proliferation and metabolism of cancer cells are now widely used to treat cancer that has spread.

Biologic Therapy

Biologic therapy is the most promising field for future developments in breast cancer therapy. Biologic therapy targets a specific feature of cancer cells, enabling the medication to attack cancer cells with little effect on normal cells. The result is less toxicity and fewer side effects, compared to other medical therapies. HER-2-positive breast cancers can now be treated with medications that selectively bind to HER-2 receptors on the cell surface. At the time of this writing, these medications include Herceptin® (trastuzumab), Kadcyla® (ado-trastuzumab emtansine), Perjeta® (pertuzumab), and Tykerb® (lapatinib), and Nerlynx™ (neratinib). As discussed above, HER-2-positive tumors previously had a relatively poor prognosis (expected outcome) compared to most breast cancers, but excellent results can now be expected with biologic therapy together with chemotherapy.

Preparing for Chemotherapy Treatments

- [ ] Eat breakfast and drink plenty of fluids before chemotherapy. Being dehydrated will make it difficult for the oncology nurse to find a vein.

- [ ] Do NOT skip taking your usual daily prescriptions, unless told otherwise by your doctor.

- [ ] Wear loose-fitting clothing so that you are comfortable while sitting for hours.

- [ ] Wear loose sleeves that can be easily rolled up if you will receive chemotherapy through an arm vein.

- [ ] Do NOT wear an undershirt or a turtleneck if you have an injection port. It is best to wear a V-neck.

- [ ] Bring a throw blanket. (Infusion centers tend to maintain a particularly low temperature, year-round.)

- [ ] Bring a pillow from home to make yourself more comfortable.

- [ ] Bring reading material or an entertainment device to keep yourself occupied for hours.

- [ ] Bring a pail or a large bag to use if you need to vomit on the way home from the treatment.

CHEMOTHERAPY AND
WOMEN OVER AGE SEVENTY

There is controversy as to whether women over age seventy should be treated with adjuvant chemotherapy (see below); as a result, some oncologists will not routinely offer chemotherapy to older women. Several factors underlie this practice. One reason is a lack of scientific data showing evidence that chemotherapy benefits older women. Because the large scientific studies published to date excluded women over seventy from their research protocols, little data exists on the success of chemotherapy with women in this age group. A second reason that chemotherapy might not be offered to older women is that the long-term benefits may be projected to occur beyond the average expected life span of the woman. In other words, it might not be considered worthwhile to subject a woman to the side effects of chemotherapy to prevent the future return of breast cancer that might not occur for many years if that woman's age already approaches her statistical life expectancy. A final reason that chemotherapy might not be offered to women over age seventy is that doctors may assume (correctly or incorrectly) that older women are likely to have multiple other health problems that might be exacerbated by chemotherapy drugs. For instance, patients with congestive heart failure cannot be treated with Adriamycin, which is toxic to heart tissue.

....

Chemotherapy

Systemic chemotherapy has long been the standard treatment for metastatic disease. Increasingly, chemotherapy is used to treat breast cancer patients with no evidence for metastases. The term *adjuvant chemotherapy* is used to describe chemotherapy given to prevent recurrence of breast cancer in patients who have had a lumpectomy or a mastectomy and do not have evidence of metastatic disease. The term *neoadjuvant therapy* is used for cancer treatment performed before surgical removal of the cancer in order to downgrade the cancer to a less severe stage preoperatively.

Neoadjuvant therapy may be done to shrink a tumor so that a patient who initially would have required a mastectomy becomes a candidate for lumpectomy. Neoadjuvant therapy may also be done to make an inoperable cancer operable. In other words, a cancer that would otherwise be considered untreatable may become eligible for treatment following successful neoadjuvant therapy. One example of this is breast cancer widely invading the ribs and muscles of the chest wall. Neoadjuvant therapy may be administered in the form of chemotherapy or hormone therapy.

Chemotherapy is generally administered in specialized infusion centers by specially trained chemotherapy nurses. These powerful drugs are given through intravenous lines over a period of hours. Patients sit in comfortable chairs, and there may be a shared television for the patients to watch. The drugs are often administered through a needle placed directly into an arm vein. Alternatively, if it's difficult to access your veins, your oncologist may recommend that you have a minor operation to implant an injection port under your skin near the collarbone. The port is composed of a reservoir shaped like a small drum, connected to an internal catheter that leads into a major vein. The port is accessed for chemotherapy by inserting a needle through the skin into the reservoir.

Chemotherapy drugs generally work by attacking cells that divide rapidly, since cancer cells divide more rapidly than most normal cells. However, certain parts of the body have healthy cells that normally divide rapidly, including the hair follicles, the lining of the digestive tract, and blood-producing cells. As a consequence, side effects of chemotherapy often include hair loss, digestive symptoms, and low blood counts. Other side effects of chemotherapy may include fatigue, loss of appetite, nausea, vomiting, and peripheral neuropathy, or damage to the nerves of the hands or feet that may result in numbness or tingling. These nerve symptoms could be either temporary or permanent. A significant side effect of some chemotherapy is the rapid onset of menopause in menstruating women. One class of chemotherapy drugs, anthracyclines, can permanently reduce the heart's ability to pump blood in a small proportion of patients. To minimize the chance of serious heart damage, patients treated with these drugs are monitored for changes in cardiac function. In addition, there is also a limit on the lifetime dose of these drugs that may be given to any patient. Doctors may treat patients undergoing chemotherapy with additional medications to treat the side effects of chemotherapy. These drugs include medications to reduce nausea and vomiting. In some cases, patients receiving chemotherapy are given Neupogen® (filgrastim) to treat falling white blood cell counts.

Chemotherapy Regimens

Chemotherapy is typically administered as a combination of multiple drugs. The drugs are combined in a manner that includes two or three agents that attack cancer cells in different ways. The preferred chemotherapy treatments for HER-2-negative breast cancer are dose-dense AC (Adriamycin® and cyclophosphamide), followed by paclitaxel or TC (Taxotere® and cyclophosphamide). Other, less commonly used chemotherapy regimens include CMF (cyclophosphamide, methotrexate, and fluorouracil), EC (epirubicin and cyclophosphamide), and TAC (Taxotere, Adriamycin, and cyclophosphamide). Alternatively, AC may be given in a regimen that is not dose-dense and followed by cycles of docetaxel or paclitaxel.

Chemotherapy is typically given in treatment cycles alternating with periods of rest. These breaks provide the intestinal lining and other sensitive parts of the body with an opportunity to recover from the toxic effects of chemotherapy. *Dose-dense* chemotherapy is the term used to describe chemotherapy treatments that are given on a more frequent schedule than traditional cycles. For instance, the original regimen for AC comprised four cycles of AC administered once every twenty-one days. By contrast, dose-dense AC comprises four cycles of AC administered once every fourteen days.

Oncologists often treat cancer according to a set of guidelines that are published by the National Comprehensive Cancer Network (NCCN) and updated periodically. Other guideline agencies exist, and guidelines are sometimes controversial, depending on the quality of the studies that are used to develop them. These guidelines include very specific flowcharts outlining the appropriate therapy for nearly every conceivable combination of breast cancer features. These guidelines are based on scientific data, and provide for uniformity of treatment by different doctors in big cities and small towns across the United States. You can ask your oncologist to show you the NCCN flowchart that corresponds to your specific cancer and your treatment. If your doctor is not familiar with these flowcharts, you can let him or her know that the flowcharts are available to doctors online, at no cost, at *https://www.nccn.org/professionals/physician_gls/default.aspx#site*. You should keep in mind the fact that the NCCN flowcharts may not always be 100 percent up to date. If your oncologist follows the latest developments in cancer research, he or she may offer you a treatment that has not yet been included in the official guidelines. In addition, it is possible that you will be offered an opportunity to participate in a research study, and receive an experimental treatment. Taking part in these studies can sometimes be a chance to receive tomorrow's miracle drug, today.

Notes

_____
_____
_____
_____
_____
_____
_____
_____
_____
_____
_____
_____
_____
_____
_____
_____
_____
_____
_____
_____
_____
_____
_____
_____
_____
_____

CHAPTER 9

Reconstructive & Cosmetic Breast Surgery

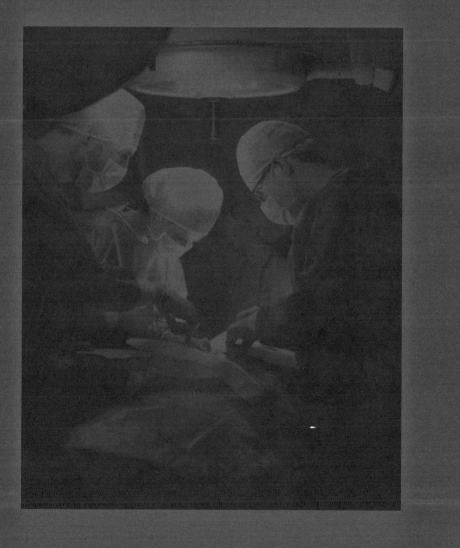

9

Reconstructive & Cosmetic Breast Surgery

Questions to Ask Your Surgeon before Breast Reconstruction Surgery

☐ Will I need more than one surgery? How many operations should I expect?

☐ Will I have an overnight hospital stay?

☐ Will a tissue expander be implanted to stretch the skin? (A tissue expander is like a collapsed beach ball that is implanted temporarily and injected with saline solution over a period of weeks.) How many visits will I need to achieve full expansion? Will I need surgery to replace the expander with a permanent breast implant?

☐ Will I need surgery on the healthy breast to make the two breasts symmetrical?

☐ Will I have nipple reconstruction? How will the new nipple be created?

☐ If there will be flap reconstruction—using tissue from elsewhere on my body to rebuild the breast—where will the flap come from? Where will the scars be?

PLASTIC SURGERY HAS BEEN AN OFFICIALLY RECOGNIZED SPECIALTY since 1941. This field includes two major categories of surgery: reconstructive and cosmetic. Reconstructive surgery is performed to correct deformities resulting from birth defects, injuries, or major surgery. Cosmetic surgery is performed to improve the patient's appearance, and can sometimes result in an enormous improvement in a person's quality of life. A large proportion of both the reconstructive and cosmetic surgeries performed in the United States involve the breasts. According to statistics from the American Society for Aesthetic Plastic Surgery, breast augmentation and breast lift were among the five cosmetic surgery procedures performed most frequently in the United States during 2016.

Breast Reconstruction Surgery

BREAST RECONSTRUCTION SURGERY IS PERFORMED TO GIVE A WOMAN the appearance of having two breasts following a mastectomy. Research has indicated that breast reconstruction has psychosocial benefits for women undergoing mastectomy and results in improved quality of life, compared to women who have mastectomy without reconstruction. For this reason, a federal law was passed in 1998—the Women's Health and Cancer Rights Act—mandating that health insurance plans must cover breast reconstruction surgery. Despite this coverage, fewer than 20 percent of women undergoing mastectomy in the United States elect to have breast reconstruction surgery. Breast reconstruction may include a breast implant, or may be done entirely with the patient's own living tissue, taken from another part of the body. Since breast skin is removed, along with the mammary gland, during a standard mastectomy, there may be too little skin left to cover a full-sized breast implant. In this case, a tissue expander may be placed at the mastectomy site before inserting a breast implant. The tissue expander is like an uninflated beach ball. The skin will heal over the expander and a scar forms at the mastectomy site. Over multiple visits, the surgeon will inject saline solution (salt water) through the skin into the tissue expander. As the expander gradually inflates, the skin over it will stretch until there is enough space for the surgeon to perform an exchange operation and insert a breast implant in place of the tissue expander.

Natural tissue from other parts of the body may be used for breast reconstruction surgery, and may come from the abdomen, the buttock, or the flank (the side region of the torso near the kidneys). For a slim woman, reconstruction with breast implants is usually the only option. If a woman is overweight and desires breast reconstruction, then using excess tissue from her own body may be an option. In fact, taking tissue from the abdomen or buttocks may result in an additional benefit of reducing a region with excess fat. Two reconstruction operations involve rotating tissue from the torso into the position of the breasts, while that tissue retains its original connection to its blood supply. These two procedures are the TRAM flap (TRAM stands for transverse rectus abdominis), which utilizes tissue from the abdomen, and the latissimus flap, which uses tissue from the flank. In the TRAM flap procedure, the surgeon takes a large ellipse of tissue from the front of the abdomen in the vicinity of the belt line. The tissue includes skin, subcutaneous fat, and the underlying muscle. One end of the muscle retains its original connection to the body, providing a blood supply for the reconstructed breast. The ellipse of tissue that is removed from the abdomen can be used to simultaneously reconstruct two breasts, in the case of a double mastectomy. However, if only one breast is reconstructed at the time of the TRAM flap, there will be no possibility in the future of performing a second TRAM flap procedure for the second breast.

In contrast to the TRAM flap and the latissimus flap, the gluteus free flap reconstruction does not leave the vessels connected. Tissue from the buttock, including skin, subcutaneous fat, and underlying muscle, is completely separated from the body and transplanted to the mastectomy site. Reattaching the tissue requires microsurgery to attach blood vessels to the reconstructed breast. This can be a more challenging operation, and not all plastic surgeons are experienced in microsurgery techniques.

The presence of a nipple and areola is a key feature in giving the reconstructed tissue the identity of a breast. Therefore, breast reconstruction surgery usually includes creation of a nipple. A three-dimensional nipple can be created with tissue transplanted from elsewhere in the body, or a two-dimensional image of a nipple and areola can be tattooed onto the skin of the reconstructed breast to simulate the appearance of a nipple.

Surgery to Make the Breasts Symmetrical

When a plastic surgeon performs breast reconstruction surgery, it is often not possible for the surgeon to make the reconstructed breast perfectly match the opposite breast. In order to have the best overall cosmetic appearance of the whole chest, as well as symmetry of the two breasts, it is common for the surgeon to operate on the opposite healthy breast as well as the side of the mastectomy. For instance, if a woman with sagging breasts has a mastectomy and reconstruction utilizing a breast implant, the reconstructed breast may be dome-shaped and contrast sharply with the drooping opposite breast. In such cases, the surgeon may perform a breast lift (mastopexy) on the opposite breast, inserting a breast implant to match the appearance of the other side. The Women's Health and Cancer Rights Act of 1998 mandated that health insurance plans in the United States cover cosmetic surgery on the opposite breast to create a symmetrical appearance of the breasts following cancer surgery. Whether this is breast reduction or augmentation with a breast implant, insurance companies are required to cover the surgery.

Cosmetic Breast Enlargement Surgery

SURGICAL BREAST ENLARGEMENT (IN MEDICAL TERMINOLOGY, *augmentation mammoplasty*) is achieved by implanting a space-occupying object inside the breast. The presence of this breast implant increases the volume of the breast. Following the surgical placement of the implant, the skin of the breast must stretch. The incision is usually made along the border of the areola (the pigmented circle surrounding the nipple) so that the scar will hardly be noticeable. Other possible incision sites include along the armpit, or beneath the breast, along the margin where the breast meets the torso. The implant consists of a thin capsule that is about the size of a sandwich bag. This tough capsule is filled either with silicone gel or with saline solution (salt water). The implant can be surgically inserted either in front of the pectoralis muscle (between the mammary gland and the muscle) or behind the pectoralis muscle (between the muscle and the ribs). Silicone implants feel more like natural breast tissue. By contrast, some women with saline implants sometimes feel like there is sloshing water in their breasts when they make abrupt movements.

Questions to Ask Yourself If You Are Considering Breast Enlargement Surgery

☐ Are you considering surgery to please yourself, or to please someone else?

☐ Have you tried wearing a bra designed to make your breasts appear larger?

☐ Have you considered the impact that breast implants have on future screening for breast cancer?

☐ Have you considered the impact that this might have on breastfeeding in the future?

☐ Are you aware that the Food and Drug Administration recommends that breast implants be removed after ten years?

Considerations

Before considering getting breast implants, it is important to consider several consequences of this choice.

Cost and health risks. Surgery is expensive and the recovery is painful. Furthermore, all surgery and general anesthesia carry real risks to your health and   g an incision around the areola is loss of nipple sensation. Other recognized complications include permanently erect nipples and the inability to breastfeed. If you are contemplating breast enlargement surgery and plan to breastfeed, this is an important issue to discuss with your surgeon. Careful surgical planning can maximize the chance that breastfeeding will be possible in the future. One long-term complication of breast implants that may occur years after the augmentation surgery is that the body may treat the implant as a foreign body and develop a reaction to it. A similar reaction occurs when an oyster reacts to an irritating particle of sand that is trapped within its shell by depositing layers of mother-of-pearl over the particle, resulting in a smooth, hard pearl. In a similar manner, the human body may deposit calcium around a breast implant. This complication is more common in implants that are located in front of the pectoralis muscle than in implants behind the muscle. If the body deposits a significant amount of calcium around the implant, the implant may become rock-hard. The only treatment for this complication is to remove the implant and the stony calcified capsule.

Implants and breast cancer screening. The consequence of breast augmentation that I most commonly face in my own practice is difficulty screening women with implants for breast cancer. For example, the presence of the implant makes it much more difficult to feel a lump in the breast. Mammograms are routinely performed on women with breast implants. However, in order to visualize the most breast tissue possible, twice as many images must be obtained, compared to mammography on women who do not have breast implants. Even on properly performed mammograms, a portion of the breast is always obscured by the breast implant, which could possibly hide a breast cancer.

Removal and replacement. The FDA (Food and Drug Administration) recommends that breast implants be removed after ten years. No breast implant is expected to last forever, and breast implants sometimes rupture. Different problems may arise, depending on whether the material that leaks out of a breast implant is saline solution or silicone gel. When a saline breast implant ruptures, the body rapidly absorbs the saline solution and the capsule completely collapses, becoming nearly flat over a period of a few days. If the woman wants to have the collapsed implant replaced with a new implant, which is commonly the case, this surgery should be done quickly. If the ruptured saline implant remains collapsed for too long, the body will close the space in the breast that held the original implant. If there is no longer a space large enough to hold a replacement implant, the cosmetic surgeon will need to perform a more involved operation to insert a new implant.

Alternatively, when a silicone breast implant ruptures, free silicone gel may be released into the breast. A number of patients with ruptured silicone breast implants previously claimed that the silicone gel released into their breasts caused serious health problems, and they filed class action lawsuits against the manufacturers. As a consequence of these lawsuits, there was limited availability of silicone breast implants in the United States between 1992 and 2006. Since there is no compelling evidence in the scientific literature that ruptured silicone breast implants cause health problems, silicone breast implants have become widely available once again.

Personal motivations. If you are considering breast augmentation surgery, it is important to honestly assess your true motivation. If you are considering breast augmentation because you don't like the way you look in clothes, try different style choices. Alternatively, you might consider trying a padded bra or a push-up bra to create the illusion of larger breasts.

Many women undergo breast enlargement to solve problems that, in reality, are not rooted in their breast size. For instance, some women endure breast augmentation surgery because they believe that it will give them greater self-confidence. There are much better ways to improve self-image than through cosmetic surgery, and these alternatives deserve serious investigation. Other women consider having breast augmentation to save their marriage (or another relationship), which is not likely to be fixed by surgery. Couples counseling is much more likely to have a long-lasting positive impact on a relationship. Finally, if anyone pressures you to have cosmetic surgery, remember that it is your body, and if you are happy with your body, you should think carefully before you go through surgery to make somebody else happy. A good exercise is to ask yourself if you would ever ask anybody you love to go through elective surgery to make *you* happy.

Nonsurgical Options

Some women seek means of breast enlargement besides surgery. Wearing padded bras and placing inserts into oversized bras are effective solutions. These space-occupying inserts are available in silicone, polyurethane foam rubber, and other materials. Schemes claiming to achieve "breast enlargement" through exercise are deceptive. It is certainly possible to build up the pectoralis muscles through exercise. However, a quick look at images of the winners of women's bodybuilding contests will make it clear that building large pectoralis muscles does not increase the size of the breasts.

Breast enlargement schemes other than breast implants and padded bras are generally scams. Some of these schemes, such as certain herbs and supplements, are a harmless waste of money. Other schemes are dangerous and could cause lifelong health problems. Harmful breast enlargement schemes often involve injecting foreign materials into the breast. Assorted quacks and practitioners have tried injecting silicone, paraffin wax, cooking oil, and fat into women's breasts. None of these injections are likely to have satisfactory results. Complications are frequent and include infection, allergic reactions, forming of scar tissue as a reaction to foreign bodies, extreme lumpiness, and potentially fatal embolism (particles traveling through the bloodstream). Migration of these foreign materials is common, since there is no natural barrier within the breast to keep the free foreign substance in one place. The effect of gravity may cause the injected material to migrate beyond the breast toward the waist.

Breast Reduction Surgery

BREAST REDUCTION SURGERY IS OFTEN CONSIDERED when the breasts are so large and heavy that the patient experiences chronic back pain. Breast reduction may also be considered when a woman has difficulty finding clothing that fits her comfortably and looks flattering. Finally, women with large breasts may be self-conscious about their appearance or may become victims of sexual harassment.

Questions to Ask Yourself If You Are Considering Breast Reduction Surgery

- ☐ If you are overweight, have you made a serious effort to lose weight?
- ☐ Have you tried wearing a minimizer bra, designed to make your breasts appear smaller?
- ☐ Have you tried wearing a bra with wide, comfortable straps and maximum support to reduce strain on your shoulders?
- ☐ Have you considered the impact that this surgery might have on breastfeeding in the future?

Considerations

Breast reduction is an extensive operation that must be carefully planned to have a natural-appearing result, with the nipple located in the correct position. This surgery almost always leaves a large, anchor-shaped scar. The scar forms a circle around the nipple and extends in a straight vertical line to the bottom of the breast. At its lower end, the straight scar meets the center of an arc-shaped scar along the bottom margin of the breast (where the breast meets the torso). Women who undergo breast reduction surgery usually are unable to breastfeed their infants. Possible complications include infection and formation of a thick, shiny, raised (keloid) scar. Women who have a tendency to form keloid scars are at the greatest risk for this complication, and should discuss options with their plastic surgeon, who may take steps to reduce the likelihood of this unwanted outcome.

Alternatives to Surgery

As with breast enlargement, buying the right bra may be a viable alternative to surgery for some women. There are minimizer bras designed to allow a woman with large breasts to wear clothing designed for women with smaller breasts. Many women who contemplate breast reduction complain of problems with their back and shoulders, resulting from the weight of their breasts. These women might benefit from switching to a bra that provides more support or has wider shoulder straps. In the majority of cases, women who believe they would benefit from breast reduction surgery are overweight. For these women, it is a worthwhile exercise to undertake a serious weight reduction program before committing to the pain and expense of breast reduction surgery. For many overweight women contemplating breast reduction surgery, losing weight would have multiple benefits, including decreased breast size, improved blood pressure, reversal of pre-diabetes, and a slimmer appearance. Admittedly, "lose weight" is easy advice to give, but very difficult to achieve.

Breast Lift

THE TERM *BREAST LIFT* (MASTOPEXY) IS USED TO DESCRIBE a diverse group of procedures for the treatment of drooping breasts, including, on the one hand, variations of breast reduction surgery and, on the other hand, the use of breast implants. Breast lift candidates include patients with excessive loose skin over the breasts and women whose breasts sag to a degree that the nipples are located significantly below the inframammary fold (the line at the bottom margin of the breast where the breast joins the torso). If you are contemplating a surgical breast lift, it is important to ask your surgeon for a detailed explanation of exactly what the surgery will entail (see the checklist below).

I have met a number of patients in my practice who have had breast lifts, but are unaware that their surgeon performed an operation that included placing implants in each breast. As with other types of cosmetic breast surgery, women considering a breast lift would be wise to first try purchasing a bra that will give them superior support and keep their breasts from sagging.

Questions to Ask Your Surgeon
If You Are Considering Breast Lift Surgery

- [ ] Do you plan to remove breast tissue?
- [ ] Will my bra size be smaller following recovery from the surgery?
- [ ] Do you intend to put implants in the breasts?
- [ ] Where will the scars be located?
- [ ] Do you plan to change the location of the nipple?
- [ ] Will this surgery impact my ability to breastfeed in the future?

Nipple Surgery

NIPPLE INVERSION OCCURS WHEN A NIPPLE DOES NOT PROJECT from the breast, but instead is pulled in, below the level of the surrounding areola. Nipple inversion can be an important symptom, indicating the presence of breast cancer. A malignant (cancerous) tumor in the breast can exert traction on the nipple, pulling it inward. However, not all nipple inversion is caused by cancer. Some women have had a retracted nipple for many years, and mammography shows no evidence of breast cancer. If a woman is self-conscious about the presence of an inverted nipple, and a doctor has determined that it is not the result of breast cancer, it is possible to have a nipple-release procedure performed by a plastic surgeon. This operation can result in a normal-appearing nipple. It is important to be aware that women with inverted nipples are usually capable of nursing their babies normally, but women who have had a nipple-release procedure are usually not able to breastfeed.

Some women choose to have their nipples pierced so that they can wear jewelry on their nipples. This practice does not result in increased risk of breast cancer, but it is important for the procedure to be performed with careful attention to sterile technique so that it does not cause an infection. Women who consider nipple piercing should bear in mind that this could potentially result in scarring of the milk ducts, which might interfere with breastfeeding in the future.

Notes

Notes

Mammogram Results

Mammogram Results

APPOINTMENT DATE	DOCTOR
6 / 15/ 18	Dr. Fowler

FACILITY NAME	PHONE
Cedars-Sinai	212-555-4567

RESULTS: ☑ NORMAL   ☐ ABNORMAL

BREAST DENSITY: ☐ DENSE   ☑ NOT DENSE

SCHEDULE NEXT APPOINTMENT IN:

☐ 6 MONTHS   ☑ 1 YEAR   ☐ 2 YEARS

RECOMMENDED FOLLOW-UP TESTS:

☑ NO ADDITIONAL TESTS RECOMMENDED

☐ BREAST ULTRASOUND   ☐ BREAST MRI   ☐ OTHER _____

NOTES: send disk of prior mammograms to radiologist

SAMPLE

APPOINTMENT DATE

DOCTOR

FACILITY NAME

PHONE

RESULTS: ☐ NORMAL ☐ ABNORMAL

BREAST DENSITY: ☐ DENSE ☐ NOT DENSE

SCHEDULE NEXT APPOINTMENT IN:
☐ 6 MONTHS ☐ 1 YEAR ☐ 2 YEARS

RECOMMENDED FOLLOW-UP TESTS:
☐ NO ADDITIONAL TESTS RECOMMENDED
☐ BREAST ULTRASOUND ☐ BREAST MRI ☐ OTHER_____

NOTES:

APPOINTMENT DATE

DOCTOR

FACILITY NAME

PHONE

RESULTS: ☐ NORMAL ☐ ABNORMAL

BREAST DENSITY: ☐ DENSE ☐ NOT DENSE

SCHEDULE NEXT APPOINTMENT IN:
☐ 6 MONTHS ☐ 1 YEAR ☐ 2 YEARS

RECOMMENDED FOLLOW-UP TESTS:
☐ NO ADDITIONAL TESTS RECOMMENDED
☐ BREAST ULTRASOUND ☐ BREAST MRI ☐ OTHER_____

NOTES:

APPOINTMENT DATE   **DOCTOR**

FACILITY NAME   **PHONE**

RESULTS: ☐ NORMAL   ☐ ABNORMAL

BREAST DENSITY: ☐ DENSE   ☐ NOT DENSE

SCHEDULE NEXT APPOINTMENT IN:
☐ 6 MONTHS   ☐ 1 YEAR   ☐ 2 YEARS

RECOMMENDED FOLLOW-UP TESTS:
☐ NO ADDITIONAL TESTS RECOMMENDED
☐ BREAST ULTRASOUND   ☐ BREAST MRI   ☐ OTHER_____

NOTES:

APPOINTMENT DATE   **DOCTOR**

FACILITY NAME   **PHONE**

RESULTS: ☐ NORMAL   ☐ ABNORMAL

BREAST DENSITY: ☐ DENSE   ☐ NOT DENSE

SCHEDULE NEXT APPOINTMENT IN:
☐ 6 MONTHS   ☐ 1 YEAR   ☐ 2 YEARS

RECOMMENDED FOLLOW-UP TESTS:
☐ NO ADDITIONAL TESTS RECOMMENDED
☐ BREAST ULTRASOUND   ☐ BREAST MRI   ☐ OTHER_____

NOTES:

APPOINTMENT DATE   DOCTOR

FACILITY NAME   PHONE

RESULTS: ☐ NORMAL   ☐ ABNORMAL

BREAST DENSITY: ☐ DENSE   ☐ NOT DENSE

SCHEDULE NEXT APPOINTMENT IN:
☐ 6 MONTHS   ☐ 1 YEAR   ☐ 2 YEARS

RECOMMENDED FOLLOW-UP TESTS:
☐ NO ADDITIONAL TESTS RECOMMENDED
☐ BREAST ULTRASOUND   ☐ BREAST MRI   ☐ OTHER_____

NOTES:

APPOINTMENT DATE   DOCTOR

FACILITY NAME   PHONE

RESULTS: ☐ NORMAL   ☐ ABNORMAL

BREAST DENSITY: ☐ DENSE   ☐ NOT DENSE

SCHEDULE NEXT APPOINTMENT IN:
☐ 6 MONTHS   ☐ 1 YEAR   ☐ 2 YEARS

RECOMMENDED FOLLOW-UP TESTS:
☐ NO ADDITIONAL TESTS RECOMMENDED
☐ BREAST ULTRASOUND   ☐ BREAST MRI   ☐ OTHER_____

NOTES:

APPOINTMENT DATE   **DOCTOR**

FACILITY NAME   **PHONE**

RESULTS: ☐ NORMAL   ☐ ABNORMAL

BREAST DENSITY: ☐ DENSE   ☐ NOT DENSE

SCHEDULE NEXT APPOINTMENT IN:
☐ 6 MONTHS   ☐ 1 YEAR   ☐ 2 YEARS

RECOMMENDED FOLLOW-UP TESTS:
☐ NO ADDITIONAL TESTS RECOMMENDED
☐ BREAST ULTRASOUND   ☐ BREAST MRI   ☐ OTHER_____

NOTES:

APPOINTMENT DATE   **DOCTOR**

FACILITY NAME   **PHONE**

RESULTS: ☐ NORMAL   ☐ ABNORMAL

BREAST DENSITY: ☐ DENSE   ☐ NOT DENSE

SCHEDULE NEXT APPOINTMENT IN:
☐ 6 MONTHS   ☐ 1 YEAR   ☐ 2 YEARS

RECOMMENDED FOLLOW-UP TESTS:
☐ NO ADDITIONAL TESTS RECOMMENDED
☐ BREAST ULTRASOUND   ☐ BREAST MRI   ☐ OTHER_____

NOTES:

APPOINTMENT DATE   DOCTOR

FACILITY NAME   PHONE

RESULTS: ☐ NORMAL   ☐ ABNORMAL

BREAST DENSITY: ☐ DENSE   ☐ NOT DENSE

SCHEDULE NEXT APPOINTMENT IN:
☐ 6 MONTHS   ☐ 1 YEAR   ☐ 2 YEARS

RECOMMENDED FOLLOW-UP TESTS:
☐ NO ADDITIONAL TESTS RECOMMENDED
☐ BREAST ULTRASOUND   ☐ BREAST MRI   ☐ OTHER_____

NOTES:

APPOINTMENT DATE   DOCTOR

FACILITY NAME   PHONE

RESULTS: ☐ NORMAL   ☐ ABNORMAL

BREAST DENSITY: ☐ DENSE   ☐ NOT DENSE

SCHEDULE NEXT APPOINTMENT IN:
☐ 6 MONTHS   ☐ 1 YEAR   ☐ 2 YEARS

RECOMMENDED FOLLOW-UP TESTS:
☐ NO ADDITIONAL TESTS RECOMMENDED
☐ BREAST ULTRASOUND   ☐ BREAST MRI   ☐ OTHER_____

NOTES:

Notes

Breast Ultrasound & MRI Results

Breast Ultrasound Results

APPOINTMENT DATE	DOCTOR
10 / 1/ 18	Dr. Smith

FACILITY NAME	PHONE
Cedars-Sinai	212-555-4567

RESULTS: ☑ NORMAL ☐ ABNORMAL

SCHEDULE NEXT APPOINTMENT IN:

☐ NO FOLLOW-UP APPNT. NEEDED ☐ 6 MONTHS ☑ OTHER *tomorrow*

RECOMMENDED FOLLOW-UP TESTS:

☐ NONE ☐ MAMMOGRAM
☑ BREAST MRI ☐ ULTRASOUND-GUIDED BIOPSY

NOTES: complicated cyst

SAMPLE

APPOINTMENT DATE   **DOCTOR**

FACILITY NAME   **PHONE**

RESULTS: ☐ NORMAL   ☐ ABNORMAL

SCHEDULE NEXT APPOINTMENT IN:
☐ NO FOLLOW-UP APPNT. NEEDED   ☐ 6 MONTHS   ☐ OTHER _____

RECOMMENDED FOLLOW-UP TESTS:
☐ NONE   ☐ MAMMOGRAM
☐ BREAST MRI   ☐ ULTRASOUND-GUIDED BIOPSY

NOTES:
_____
_____
_____
_____

APPOINTMENT DATE   **DOCTOR**

FACILITY NAME   **PHONE**

RESULTS: ☐ NORMAL   ☐ ABNORMAL

SCHEDULE NEXT APPOINTMENT IN:
☐ NO FOLLOW-UP APPNT. NEEDED   ☐ 6 MONTHS   ☐ OTHER _____

RECOMMENDED FOLLOW-UP TESTS:
☐ NONE   ☐ MAMMOGRAM
☐ BREAST MRI   ☐ ULTRASOUND-GUIDED BIOPSY

NOTES:
_____
_____
_____
_____

Breast Ultrasound Results

APPOINTMENT DATE   DOCTOR

FACILITY NAME   PHONE

RESULTS: ☐ NORMAL   ☐ ABNORMAL

SCHEDULE NEXT APPOINTMENT IN:
☐ NO FOLLOW-UP APPNT. NEEDED   ☐ 6 MONTHS ☐ OTHER _____

RECOMMENDED FOLLOW-UP TESTS:
☐ NONE   ☐ MAMMOGRAM
☐ BREAST MRI   ☐ ULTRASOUND-GUIDED BIOPSY

NOTES:

APPOINTMENT DATE   DOCTOR

FACILITY NAME   PHONE

RESULTS: ☐ NORMAL   ☐ ABNORMAL

SCHEDULE NEXT APPOINTMENT IN:
☐ NO FOLLOW-UP APPNT. NEEDED   ☐ 6 MONTHS ☐ OTHER _____

RECOMMENDED FOLLOW-UP TESTS:
☐ NONE   ☐ MAMMOGRAM
☐ BREAST MRI   ☐ ULTRASOUND-GUIDED BIOPSY

NOTES:

Breast Ultrasound Results

APPOINTMENT DATE   **DOCTOR**

FACILITY NAME   **PHONE**

RESULTS: ☐ NORMAL   ☐ ABNORMAL

SCHEDULE NEXT APPOINTMENT IN:
☐ NO FOLLOW-UP APPNT. NEEDED   ☐ 6 MONTHS   ☐ OTHER _____

RECOMMENDED FOLLOW-UP TESTS:
☐ NONE   ☐ MAMMOGRAM
☐ BREAST MRI   ☐ ULTRASOUND-GUIDED BIOPSY

NOTES:

APPOINTMENT DATE   **DOCTOR**

FACILITY NAME   **PHONE**

RESULTS: ☐ NORMAL   ☐ ABNORMAL

SCHEDULE NEXT APPOINTMENT IN:
☐ NO FOLLOW-UP APPNT. NEEDED   ☐ 6 MONTHS   ☐ OTHER _____

RECOMMENDED FOLLOW-UP TESTS:
☐ NONE   ☐ MAMMOGRAM
☐ BREAST MRI   ☐ ULTRASOUND-GUIDED BIOPSY

NOTES:

Breast Ultrasound Results

APPOINTMENT DATE

DOCTOR

FACILITY NAME

PHONE

RESULTS: ☐ NORMAL ☐ ABNORMAL

SCHEDULE NEXT APPOINTMENT IN:
☐ NO FOLLOW-UP APPNT. NEEDED ☐ 6 MONTHS ☐ OTHER _____

RECOMMENDED FOLLOW-UP TESTS:
☐ NONE ☐ MAMMOGRAM
☐ BREAST MRI ☐ ULTRASOUND-GUIDED BIOPSY

NOTES:
_____
_____
_____
_____

APPOINTMENT DATE

DOCTOR

FACILITY NAME

PHONE

RESULTS: ☐ NORMAL ☐ ABNORMAL

SCHEDULE NEXT APPOINTMENT IN:
☐ NO FOLLOW-UP APPNT. NEEDED ☐ 6 MONTHS ☐ OTHER _____

RECOMMENDED FOLLOW-UP TESTS:
☐ NONE ☐ MAMMOGRAM
☐ BREAST MRI ☐ ULTRASOUND-GUIDED BIOPSY

NOTES:
_____
_____
_____
_____

Breast Ultrasound Results

APPOINTMENT DATE   **DOCTOR**

FACILITY NAME   **PHONE**

RESULTS: ☐ NORMAL   ☐ ABNORMAL

SCHEDULE NEXT APPOINTMENT IN:
☐ NO FOLLOW-UP APPNT. NEEDED   ☐ 6 MONTHS   ☐ OTHER _____

RECOMMENDED FOLLOW-UP TESTS:
☐ NONE   ☐ MAMMOGRAM
☐ BREAST MRI   ☐ ULTRASOUND-GUIDED BIOPSY

NOTES:
_____
_____
_____
_____

APPOINTMENT DATE   **DOCTOR**

FACILITY NAME   **PHONE**

RESULTS: ☐ NORMAL   ☐ ABNORMAL

SCHEDULE NEXT APPOINTMENT IN:
☐ NO FOLLOW-UP APPNT. NEEDED   ☐ 6 MONTHS   ☐ OTHER _____

RECOMMENDED FOLLOW-UP TESTS:
☐ NONE   ☐ MAMMOGRAM
☐ BREAST MRI   ☐ ULTRASOUND-GUIDED BIOPSY

NOTES:
_____
_____
_____
_____

Breast MRI
Results

APPOINTMENT DATE	DOCTOR
10 / 1/ 18	Dr. Smith
FACILITY NAME	**PHONE**
Cedars-Sinai	212-555-4567

RESULTS: ☐ NORMAL ☑ ABNORMAL

RECOMMENDED FOLLOW-UP:
☐ NO FOLLOW-UP MRI NEEDED ☑ 6-MONTH FOLLOW-UP ☐ BIOPSY

NOTES:

left breast gadolinium uptake, probably benign

SAMPLE

APPOINTMENT DATE	DOCTOR
FACILITY NAME	**PHONE**

RESULTS: ☐ NORMAL ☐ ABNORMAL

RECOMMENDED FOLLOW-UP:
☐ NO FOLLOW-UP MRI NEEDED ☐ 6-MONTH FOLLOW-UP ☐ BIOPSY

NOTES:

APPOINTMENT DATE   DOCTOR

FACILITY NAME   PHONE

RESULTS: ☐ NORMAL   ☐ ABNORMAL

RECOMMENDED FOLLOW-UP:
☐ NO FOLLOW-UP MRI NEEDED   ☐ 6-MONTH FOLLOW-UP   ☐ BIOPSY

NOTES:

_____

_____

_____

_____

APPOINTMENT DATE   DOCTOR

FACILITY NAME   PHONE

RESULTS: ☐ NORMAL   ☐ ABNORMAL

RECOMMENDED FOLLOW-UP:
☐ NO FOLLOW-UP MRI NEEDED   ☐ 6-MONTH FOLLOW-UP   ☐ BIOPSY

NOTES:

_____

_____

_____

_____

Breast MRI Results

APPOINTMENT DATE   DOCTOR

FACILITY NAME   PHONE

RESULTS: ☐ NORMAL   ☐ ABNORMAL

RECOMMENDED FOLLOW-UP:
☐ NO FOLLOW-UP MRI NEEDED   ☐ 6-MONTH FOLLOW-UP   ☐ BIOPSY

NOTES:

_____

_____

_____

_____

APPOINTMENT DATE   DOCTOR

FACILITY NAME   PHONE

RESULTS: ☐ NORMAL   ☐ ABNORMAL

RECOMMENDED FOLLOW-UP:
☐ NO FOLLOW-UP MRI NEEDED   ☐ 6-MONTH FOLLOW-UP   ☐ BIOPSY

NOTES:

_____

_____

_____

_____

Breast MRI Results

APPOINTMENT DATE   **DOCTOR**

FACILITY NAME   **PHONE**

RESULTS: ☐ NORMAL   ☐ ABNORMAL

RECOMMENDED FOLLOW-UP:
☐ NO FOLLOW-UP MRI NEEDED   ☐ 6-MONTH FOLLOW-UP   ☐ BIOPSY

NOTES:

APPOINTMENT DATE   **DOCTOR**

FACILITY NAME   **PHONE**

RESULTS: ☐ NORMAL   ☐ ABNORMAL

RECOMMENDED FOLLOW-UP:
☐ NO FOLLOW-UP MRI NEEDED   ☐ 6-MONTH FOLLOW-UP   ☐ BIOPSY

NOTES:

Notes

Breast Biopsy Results

Breast Biopsy Results

APPOINTMENT DATE

11 / 1/ 18

DOCTOR

Dr. Smith

FACILITY NAME

Cedars-Sinai

PHONE

212-555-4567

WHICH BREAST:

left

PROCEDURE:

stereotactic biopsy

FOLLOW-UP APPOINTMENT WITH:

Dr. Smith

DATE SCHEDULED:

5 / 1/ 2019

PATHOLOGY RESULT:

benign

INSTRUCTIONS FOR AFTER-CARE:

no shower for 24 hours

PAIN-RELIEF INSTRUCTIONS (IF APPLICABLE):

NOTES:

sleep in sports bra

SAMPLE

APPOINTMENT DATE   DOCTOR

_____

FACILITY NAME   PHONE

_____

WHICH BREAST: PROCEDURE:

_____

FOLLOW-UP APPOINTMENT WITH:

_____

DATE SCHEDULED:

_____

PATHOLOGY RESULT:

_____

INSTRUCTIONS FOR AFTER-CARE:

_____

_____

_____

PAIN-RELIEF INSTRUCTIONS (IF APPLICABLE):

_____

_____

_____

NOTES:

_____

_____

_____

_____

_____

_____

_____

_____

APPOINTMENT DATE

DOCTOR

FACILITY NAME

PHONE

WHICH BREAST:

PROCEDURE:

FOLLOW-UP APPOINTMENT WITH:

DATE SCHEDULED:

PATHOLOGY RESULT:

INSTRUCTIONS FOR AFTER-CARE:

PAIN-RELIEF INSTRUCTIONS (IF APPLICABLE):

NOTES:

APPOINTMENT DATE

DOCTOR

FACILITY NAME

PHONE

WHICH BREAST:

PROCEDURE:

FOLLOW-UP APPOINTMENT WITH:

DATE SCHEDULED:

PATHOLOGY RESULT:

INSTRUCTIONS FOR AFTER-CARE:

PAIN-RELIEF INSTRUCTIONS (IF APPLICABLE):

NOTES:

APPOINTMENT DATE   DOCTOR

FACILITY NAME   PHONE

WHICH BREAST: PROCEDURE:

FOLLOW-UP APPOINTMENT WITH:

DATE SCHEDULED:

PATHOLOGY RESULT:

INSTRUCTIONS FOR AFTER-CARE:

PAIN-RELIEF INSTRUCTIONS (IF APPLICABLE):

NOTES:

APPOINTMENT DATE   DOCTOR

FACILITY NAME   PHONE

WHICH BREAST: PROCEDURE:

FOLLOW-UP APPOINTMENT WITH:

DATE SCHEDULED:

PATHOLOGY RESULT:

INSTRUCTIONS FOR AFTER-CARE:

PAIN-RELIEF INSTRUCTIONS (IF APPLICABLE):

NOTES:

Notes

Breast Cancer Treatments

Breast Cancer Treatments

Lumpectomy & Mastectomy Details

SURGERY DATE
11 / 15/ 18

SURGEON
Dr. Ortiz

FACILITY NAME
Cedars-Sinai

PHONE
212-555-4567

BREAST: ☑ LEFT ☐ RIGHT

TYPE OF OPERATION:
☑ LUMPECTOMY ☐ MASTECTOMY ☐ OTHER _____

FOLLOW-UP APPOINTMENT WITH:
Dr. Ortiz

DATE SCHEDULED:
11 / 19/ 18

INSTRUCTIONS FOR POSTSURGICAL CARE:
change dressing daily

PAIN-RELIEF INSTRUCTIONS (IF APPLICABLE):

NOTES:

SAMPLE

SURGERY DATE

SURGEON

FACILITY NAME

PHONE

BREAST: ☐ LEFT ☐ RIGHT

TYPE OF OPERATION:

☐ LUMPECTOMY ☐ MASTECTOMY ☐ OTHER _____

FOLLOW-UP APPOINTMENT WITH:

DATE SCHEDULED:

INSTRUCTIONS FOR POSTSURGICAL CARE:

PAIN-RELIEF INSTRUCTIONS (IF APPLICABLE):

NOTES:

SURGERY DATE   SURGEON

FACILITY NAME   PHONE

BREAST: ☐ LEFT   ☐ RIGHT

TYPE OF OPERATION:

☐ LUMPECTOMY   ☐ MASTECTOMY   ☐ OTHER _____

FOLLOW-UP APPOINTMENT WITH:

DATE SCHEDULED:

INSTRUCTIONS FOR POSTSURGICAL CARE:

PAIN-RELIEF INSTRUCTIONS (IF APPLICABLE):

NOTES:

Tumor Details

IS THE CANCER:

☐ DUCTAL   ☐ LOBULAR   ☐ IN SITU   ☐ IINVASIVE

WHAT IS THE SIZE OF THE TUMOR? _____ CM

IF YOU HAVE HAD A LUMPECTOMY OR AN EXCISIONAL (SURGICAL) BIOPSY, ARE THE MARGINS:

☐ POSITIVE   ☐ NEGATIVE   ☐ CLOSE

WHAT IS THE GRADE?

☐ LOW   ☐ INTERMEDIATE   ☐ HIGH

WHAT IS THE GROWTH RATE OF THE CANCER?

☐ LOW   ☐ INTERMEDIATE   ☐ HIGH

IS THE TUMOR POSITIVE FOR RECEPTORS?

☐ ESTROGEN (ER)   ☐ PROGESTERONE (PR)   ☐ HER-2

WHAT IS THE STAGE?

☐ STAGE 0 (IN SITU)   ☐ STAGE 1   ☐ STAGE 2   ☐ STAGE 3
☐ STAGE 4

NOTES:

_____

_____

_____

_____

_____

_____

Hospital Log:
Overnight Stay for Breast Surgery

SURGERY DATE
11 / 15 / 18

SURGEON
Dr. Ortiz

FACILITY NAME
Cedars-Sinai

PHONE
212-555-4567

BREAST: ☑ LEFT ☐ RIGHT

TYPE OF SURGERY: left mastectomy

MEDICINES ADMINISTERED & DOSES:

NOTES:

SAMPLE

SURGERY DATE

SURGEON

FACILITY NAME

PHONE

BREAST: ☐ LEFT ☐ RIGHT

TYPE OF SURGERY:

MEDICINES ADMINISTERED & DOSES:

NOTES:

SURGERY DATE   SURGEON

_____   _____

FACILITY NAME   PHONE

_____   _____

BREAST: ☐ LEFT   ☐ RIGHT

_____

TYPE OF SURGERY:

_____

MEDICINES ADMINISTERED & DOSES:

_____

_____

NOTES:

_____

_____

_____

SURGERY DATE   SURGEON

_____   _____

FACILITY NAME   PHONE

_____   _____

BREAST: ☐ LEFT   ☐ RIGHT

_____

TYPE OF SURGERY:

_____

MEDICINES ADMINISTERED & DOSES:

_____

_____

NOTES:

_____

_____

_____

Notes

Radiation & Chemotherapy

Radiation & Chemotherapy

Radiation Therapy Treatments

DOCTOR
Dr. Bahl

FACILITY NAME
Cedars-Sinai

PHONE
212-555-4567

BREAST: ☑ LEFT ☐ RIGHT **WAS A BOOST GIVEN?** no

ENTER THE DATES OF YOUR RADIATION THERAPY AS THEY ARE COMPLETED TO TRACK THE PROGRESS OF YOUR TREATMENT

6 / 4/ 19	6 / 5/ 19	6 / 6/ 19	6 / 7/ 19	6 / 10/ 19
6 / 11/ 19	6 / 12/ 19	6 / 13/ 19	6 / 14/ 19	6 / 17/ 19
6 / 18/ 19	6 / 19/ 19	6/ 20/ 19	6 /24/ 19	6 /25/ 19
6/26/ 19	6 /27/ 19	6 /26/ 19	6 /28/ 19	7/ 1/ 19
7/ 2/ 19	7/ 3/ 19	7/ 5/ 19		

REACTIONS:
none

NOTES:
no radiation July 4—closed for holiday

SAMPLE

DOCTOR

FACILITY NAME   PHONE

BREAST: ☐ LEFT   ☐ RIGHT   WAS A BOOST GIVEN?

ENTER THE DATES OF YOUR RADIATION THERAPY AS THEY ARE COMPLETED TO TRACK THE PROGRESS OF YOUR TREATMENT

REACTIONS:

NOTES:

Radiation Therapy Treatments

DOCTOR

FACILITY NAME   PHONE

BREAST: ☐ LEFT ☐ RIGHT   WAS A BOOST GIVEN?_____

ENTER THE DATES OF YOUR RADIATION THERAPY AS THEY ARE COMPLETED TO TRACK THE PROGRESS OF YOUR TREATMENT

REACTIONS:

_____

_____

_____

NOTES:

_____

_____

_____

_____

_____

Radiation Therapy Treatments

DOCTOR

FACILITY NAME   **PHONE**

BREAST: ☐ LEFT   ☐ RIGHT   **WAS A BOOST GIVEN?**

ENTER THE DATES OF YOUR RADIATION THERAPY AS THEY ARE COMPLETED TO
TRACK THE PROGRESS OF YOUR TREATMENT

REACTIONS:

NOTES:

Chemotherapy Treatments

DOCTOR

Dr. Bahl

FACILITY NAME

Cedars-Sinai

PHONE

212-555-4567

ENTER THE DATES OF YOUR CHEMOTHERAPY AS THEY ARE COMPLETED TO TRACK THE PROGRESS OF YOUR TREATMENT

8 / 6/ 19	8 / 9/ 19	8/20/ 19	8/23/ 19	9 / 3/ 19
9 /6/ 19				

REACTIONS:

nausea

NOTES:

SAMPLE

Chemotherapy Treatments

DOCTOR

FACILITY NAME   **PHONE**

ENTER THE DATES OF YOUR CHEMOTHERAPY AS THEY ARE COMPLETED TO TRACK
THE PROGRESS OF YOUR TREATMENT

REACTIONS:

NOTES:

Chemotherapy Treatments

DOCTOR

FACILITY NAME   **PHONE**

ENTER THE DATES OF YOUR CHEMOTHERAPY AS THEY ARE COMPLETED TO TRACK
THE PROGRESS OF YOUR TREATMENT

REACTIONS:

NOTES:

Chemotherapy Treatments

DOCTOR

FACILITY NAME   PHONE

ENTER THE DATES OF YOUR CHEMOTHERAPY AS THEY ARE COMPLETED TO TRACK
THE PROGRESS OF YOUR TREATMENT

REACTIONS:

NOTES:

Notes

Medications & Supplements

Medication List

DRUG NAME	DESCRIPTION	DAILY SCHEDULE 2X	
Lasix	white oval tablet	TIME	DOSAGE
DOCTOR	WHY	8am	4mg
Dr. Smith	water retention	5pm	4mg
SPECIAL INSTRUCTIONS			
ADVERSE REACTIONS			
DATE STARTED 6 / 18 / 18			
DATE ENDED			

SAMPLE

DRUG NAME	DESCRIPTION	DAILY SCHEDULE 1X	
Lipitor	white oval tablet	TIME	DOSAGE
DOCTOR	WHY elevated cholesterol levels	8am	10mg
Dr. Smith			
SPECIAL INSTRUCTIONS			
ADVERSE REACTIONS			
DATE STARTED 5 / 1 / 18			
DATE ENDED			

SAMPLE

Medications & Supplements

DRUG NAME	DESCRIPTION	DAILY SCHEDULE	
		TIME	DOSAGE
DOCTOR	WHY		
SPECIAL INSTRUCTIONS			
ADVERSE REACTIONS			
DATE STARTED			
DATE ENDED			

DRUG NAME	DESCRIPTION	DAILY SCHEDULE	
		TIME	DOSAGE
DOCTOR	WHY		
SPECIAL INSTRUCTIONS			
ADVERSE REACTIONS			
DATE STARTED			
DATE ENDED			

DRUG NAME	DESCRIPTION	DAILY SCHEDULE	
		TIME	DOSAGE
DOCTOR	WHY		
SPECIAL INSTRUCTIONS			
ADVERSE REACTIONS			
DATE STARTED			
DATE ENDED			

DRUG NAME	DESCRIPTION	DAILY SCHEDULE	
		TIME	DOSAGE
DOCTOR	WHY		
SPECIAL INSTRUCTIONS			
ADVERSE REACTIONS			
DATE STARTED			
DATE ENDED			

DRUG NAME	DESCRIPTION	DAILY SCHEDULE	
		TIME	DOSAGE
DOCTOR	WHY		
SPECIAL INSTRUCTIONS			
ADVERSE REACTIONS			
DATE STARTED			
DATE ENDED			

DRUG NAME	DESCRIPTION	DAILY SCHEDULE	
		TIME	DOSAGE
DOCTOR	WHY		
SPECIAL INSTRUCTIONS			
ADVERSE REACTIONS			
DATE STARTED			
DATE ENDED			

DRUG NAME	DESCRIPTION	DAILY SCHEDULE	
		TIME	DOSAGE
DOCTOR	WHY		
SPECIAL INSTRUCTIONS			
ADVERSE REACTIONS			
DATE STARTED			
DATE ENDED			

DRUG NAME	DESCRIPTION	DAILY SCHEDULE	
		TIME	DOSAGE
DOCTOR	WHY		
SPECIAL INSTRUCTIONS			
ADVERSE REACTIONS			
DATE STARTED			
DATE ENDED			

DRUG NAME	DESCRIPTION	DAILY SCHEDULE	
		TIME	DOSAGE
DOCTOR	WHY		
SPECIAL INSTRUCTIONS			
ADVERSE REACTIONS			
DATE STARTED			
DATE ENDED			

DRUG NAME	DESCRIPTION	DAILY SCHEDULE	
		TIME	DOSAGE
DOCTOR	WHY		
SPECIAL INSTRUCTIONS			
ADVERSE REACTIONS			
DATE STARTED			
DATE ENDED			

DRUG NAME	DESCRIPTION	DAILY SCHEDULE	
		TIME	DOSAGE
DOCTOR	WHY		
SPECIAL INSTRUCTIONS			
ADVERSE REACTIONS			
DATE STARTED			
DATE ENDED			

DRUG NAME	DESCRIPTION	DAILY SCHEDULE	
		TIME	DOSAGE
DOCTOR	WHY		
SPECIAL INSTRUCTIONS			
ADVERSE REACTIONS			
DATE STARTED			
DATE ENDED			

DRUG NAME	DESCRIPTION	DAILY SCHEDULE	
		TIME	DOSAGE
DOCTOR	WHY		
SPECIAL INSTRUCTIONS			
ADVERSE REACTIONS			
DATE STARTED			
DATE ENDED			

DRUG NAME	DESCRIPTION	DAILY SCHEDULE	
		TIME	DOSAGE
DOCTOR	WHY		
SPECIAL INSTRUCTIONS			
ADVERSE REACTIONS			
DATE STARTED			
DATE ENDED			

DRUG NAME	DESCRIPTION	DAILY SCHEDULE	
		TIME	DOSAGE
DOCTOR	WHY		
SPECIAL INSTRUCTIONS			
ADVERSE REACTIONS			
DATE STARTED			
DATE ENDED			

Supplement List

SUPPLEMENT NAME	DESCRIPTION	DAILY SCHEDULE 1×	
Vitamin D	yellow gel cap	TIME	DOSAGE
DOCTOR	WHY	12pm	1000 IU
N/A	bone health		
SPECIAL INSTRUCTIONS take with food			
ADVERSE REACTIONS			
DATE STARTED			
DATE ENDED			

SAMPLE

SUPPLEMENT NAME	DESCRIPTION	DAILY SCHEDULE 1×	
multivitamin	red/orange gummies	TIME	DOSAGE
DOCTOR	WHY	9am	2 gummies
N/A	N/A		
SPECIAL INSTRUCTIONS take with food			
ADVERSE REACTIONS			
DATE STARTED			
DATE ENDED			

SAMPLE

SUPPLEMENT NAME	DESCRIPTION	DAILY SCHEDULE	
		TIME	DOSAGE
DOCTOR	WHY		
SPECIAL INSTRUCTIONS			
ADVERSE REACTIONS			
DATE STARTED			
DATE ENDED			

SUPPLEMENT NAME	DESCRIPTION	DAILY SCHEDULE	
		TIME	DOSAGE
DOCTOR	WHY		
SPECIAL INSTRUCTIONS			
ADVERSE REACTIONS			
DATE STARTED			
DATE ENDED			

SUPPLEMENT NAME	DESCRIPTION	DAILY SCHEDULE	
		TIME	DOSAGE
DOCTOR	WHY		
SPECIAL INSTRUCTIONS			
ADVERSE REACTIONS			
DATE STARTED			
DATE ENDED			

SUPPLEMENT NAME	DESCRIPTION	DAILY SCHEDULE	
		TIME	DOSAGE
DOCTOR	WHY		
SPECIAL INSTRUCTIONS			
ADVERSE REACTIONS			
DATE STARTED			
DATE ENDED			

SUPPLEMENT NAME	DESCRIPTION	DAILY SCHEDULE	
		TIME	DOSAGE
DOCTOR	WHY		
SPECIAL INSTRUCTIONS			
ADVERSE REACTIONS			
DATE STARTED			
DATE ENDED			

SUPPLEMENT NAME	DESCRIPTION	DAILY SCHEDULE	
		TIME	DOSAGE
DOCTOR	WHY		
SPECIAL INSTRUCTIONS			
ADVERSE REACTIONS			
DATE STARTED			
DATE ENDED			

SUPPLEMENT NAME	DESCRIPTION	DAILY SCHEDULE	
		TIME	DOSAGE
DOCTOR	WHY		
SPECIAL INSTRUCTIONS			
ADVERSE REACTIONS			
DATE STARTED			
DATE ENDED			

SUPPLEMENT NAME	DESCRIPTION	DAILY SCHEDULE	
		TIME	DOSAGE
DOCTOR	WHY		
SPECIAL INSTRUCTIONS			
ADVERSE REACTIONS			
DATE STARTED			
DATE ENDED			

SUPPLEMENT NAME	DESCRIPTION	DAILY SCHEDULE	
		TIME	DOSAGE
DOCTOR	WHY		
SPECIAL INSTRUCTIONS			
ADVERSE REACTIONS			
DATE STARTED			
DATE ENDED			

Notes

_____

_____

_____

_____

_____

_____

_____

_____

_____

_____

_____

_____

_____

_____

_____

_____

_____

_____

_____

_____

_____

_____

_____

BREAST HEALTH DIARY

Doctors & Insurance

Doctor Contacts

DOCTOR NAME:

SPECIALTY:

TYPICAL TIME FOR ROUNDS:

OFFICE PHONE: CELL PHONE:

E-MAIL:

OFFICE RECEPTIONIST:

NURSE-PRACTITIONER: NP CONTACT INFO:

PA: PA CONTACT INFO:

HOSPITAL RESIDENT/INTERN REPORTING TO DOCTOR:

CONTACT INFO:

DOCTOR NAME:

SPECIALTY:

TYPICAL TIME FOR ROUNDS:

OFFICE PHONE: CELL PHONE:

E-MAIL:

OFFICE RECEPTIONIST:

NURSE-PRACTITIONER: NP CONTACT INFO:

PA: PA CONTACT INFO:

HOSPITAL RESIDENT/INTERN REPORTING TO DOCTOR:

CONTACT INFO:

DOCTOR NAME: _____

SPECIALTY: _____

TYPICAL TIME FOR ROUNDS: _____

OFFICE PHONE: _____ CELL PHONE: _____

E-MAIL: _____

OFFICE RECEPTIONIST: _____

NURSE-PRACTITIONER: _____ NP CONTACT INFO: _____

PA: _____ PA CONTACT INFO: _____

HOSPITAL RESIDENT/INTERN REPORTING TO DOCTOR: _____

CONTACT INFO: _____

DOCTOR NAME: _____

SPECIALTY: _____

TYPICAL TIME FOR ROUNDS: _____

OFFICE PHONE: _____ CELL PHONE: _____

E-MAIL: _____

OFFICE RECEPTIONIST: _____

NURSE-PRACTITIONER: _____ NP CONTACT INFO: _____

PA: _____ PA CONTACT INFO: _____

HOSPITAL RESIDENT/INTERN REPORTING TO DOCTOR: _____

CONTACT INFO: _____

SPECIAL NOTES: _____

_____

_____

_____

DOCTOR NAME: _____

SPECIALTY: _____

TYPICAL TIME FOR ROUNDS: _____

OFFICE PHONE: _____ CELL PHONE: _____

E-MAIL: _____

OFFICE RECEPTIONIST: _____

NURSE-PRACTITIONER: _____ NP CONTACT INFO: _____

PA: _____ PA CONTACT INFO: _____

HOSPITAL RESIDENT/INTERN REPORTING TO DOCTOR: _____

CONTACT INFO: _____

DOCTOR NAME: _____

SPECIALTY: _____

TYPICAL TIME FOR ROUNDS: _____

OFFICE PHONE: _____ CELL PHONE: _____

E-MAIL: _____

OFFICE RECEPTIONIST: _____

NURSE-PRACTITIONER: _____ NP CONTACT INFO: _____

PA: _____ PA CONTACT INFO: _____

HOSPITAL RESIDENT/INTERN REPORTING TO DOCTOR: _____

CONTACT INFO: _____

SPECIAL NOTES: _____

_____

_____

_____

DOCTOR NAME: _____

SPECIALTY: _____

TYPICAL TIME FOR ROUNDS: _____

OFFICE PHONE: _____ CELL PHONE: _____

E-MAIL: _____

OFFICE RECEPTIONIST: _____

NURSE-PRACTITIONER: _____ NP CONTACT INFO: _____

PA: _____ PA CONTACT INFO: _____

HOSPITAL RESIDENT/INTERN REPORTING TO DOCTOR: _____

CONTACT INFO: _____

DOCTOR NAME: _____

SPECIALTY: _____

TYPICAL TIME FOR ROUNDS: _____

OFFICE PHONE: _____ CELL PHONE: _____

E-MAIL: _____

OFFICE RECEPTIONIST: _____

NURSE-PRACTITIONER: _____ NP CONTACT INFO: _____

PA: _____ PA CONTACT INFO: _____

HOSPITAL RESIDENT/INTERN REPORTING TO DOCTOR: _____

CONTACT INFO: _____

SPECIAL NOTES: _____

_____

_____

_____

DOCTOR NAME: _____

SPECIALTY: _____

TYPICAL TIME FOR ROUNDS: _____

OFFICE PHONE: _____ CELL PHONE: _____

E-MAIL: _____

OFFICE RECEPTIONIST: _____

NURSE-PRACTITIONER: _____ NP CONTACT INFO: _____

PA: _____ PA CONTACT INFO: _____

HOSPITAL RESIDENT/INTERN REPORTING TO DOCTOR: _____

CONTACT INFO: _____

DOCTOR NAME: _____

SPECIALTY: _____

TYPICAL TIME FOR ROUNDS: _____

OFFICE PHONE: _____ CELL PHONE: _____

E-MAIL: _____

OFFICE RECEPTIONIST: _____

NURSE-PRACTITIONER: _____ NP CONTACT INFO: _____

PA: _____ PA CONTACT INFO: _____

HOSPITAL RESIDENT/INTERN REPORTING TO DOCTOR: _____

CONTACT INFO: _____

SPECIAL NOTES: _____

_____

_____

_____

DOCTOR NAME: _____

SPECIALTY: _____

TYPICAL TIME FOR ROUNDS: _____

OFFICE PHONE: _____ CELL PHONE: _____

E-MAIL: _____

OFFICE RECEPTIONIST: _____

NURSE-PRACTITIONER: _____ NP CONTACT INFO: _____

PA: _____ PA CONTACT INFO: _____

HOSPITAL RESIDENT/INTERN REPORTING TO DOCTOR: _____

CONTACT INFO: _____

DOCTOR NAME: _____

SPECIALTY: _____

TYPICAL TIME FOR ROUNDS: _____

OFFICE PHONE: _____ CELL PHONE: _____

E-MAIL: _____

OFFICE RECEPTIONIST: _____

NURSE-PRACTITIONER: _____ NP CONTACT INFO: _____

PA: _____ PA CONTACT INFO: _____

HOSPITAL RESIDENT/INTERN REPORTING TO DOCTOR: _____

CONTACT INFO: _____

SPECIAL NOTES: _____
_____
_____
_____

PRIMARY INSURANCE

INSURANCE COMPANY

NAME OF POLICY HOLDER   DATE OF BIRTH

GROUP PLAN NUMBER

MEMBER ID NUMBER:

CLAIMS DEPARTMENT PHONE NUMBER:

CLAIMS DEPARTMENT MAILING ADDRESS

SECONDARY INSURANCE

INSURANCE COMPANY

NAME OF POLICY HOLDER   DATE OF BIRTH

GROUP/PLAN NUMBER

MEMBER ID NUMBER

CLAIMS DEPARTMENT PHONE NUMBER

CLAIMS DEPARTMENT MAILING ADDRESS

OTHER INSURANCE

INSURANCE COMPANY

NAME OF POLICY HOLDER   DATE OF BIRTH

GROUP/PLAN NUMBER

MEMBER ID NUMBER

CLAIMS DEPARTMENT PHONE NUMBER

CLAIMS DEPARTMENT MAILING ADDRESS

PRESCRIPTION DRUG PLAN

INSURANCE COMPANY

MEMBER ID NUMBER

OTHER NUMBER FROM CARD

Notes

Notes

Notes

Acknowledgments

I AM GRATEFUL TO MY DAUGHTER, DEBORAH STACK, for convincing me to write this book. I would like to thank my editor, Meredith Hale. I have great respect for her editing skill, and I appreciate her fine judgment and hard work. Thank you to Sterling Publishing Co., Inc., especially to Barbara Berger and the art department, and to Melanie Madden and copy editor Diana Drew. I am appreciative to Steven Vogl, MD, for reviewing the section on chemotherapy. Thank you to my wife, Connie, for her patience and encouragement, as well as to my sons Walter and David for their support.

Glossary

Areola: The circle of pigmented skin surrounding the nipple. The areola may be pink or brown depending on a woman's complexion.

Aromatase inhibitor: Medication used to lower the level of estrogen in the bloodstream. Aromatase inhibitors are used primarily in postmenopausal women.

Asymmetry: Inequality of comparable structures on the right and left side of the body that would ordinarily be mirror images.

Axillary lymph node dissection: Surgery to remove all (or most) of the lymph nodes from an armpit.

Benign: Not cancerous

Bilateral: Involving both sides of the body. For example, bilateral mastectomy is removal of both the right breast and the left breast.

Biologic therapy: Targets a specific feature of cancer cells, enabling the medication to attack cancer cells with little effect on normal cells.

Brachytherapy: Radiation therapy that is accomplished by placing a radioactive source inside the body to treat cancer.

BRCA gene mutation: An abnormality in the DNA that may result in illness.

Breast imaging: Medical examinations that yield images of the inside of the breast to evaluate for abnormal conditions such as cancer. Breast imaging modalities include mammography, MRI, and ultrasound.

Breast implant: Medical prosthesis consisting of a tough bag filled with silicone gel or saline solution (salt water) that is placed in the breast, either to increase breast size (breast augmentation) or to recreate the appearance of a normal breast following mastectomy.

Breast reconstruction: Surgery to recreate the appearance of a natural breast following mastectomy. This term is also used to refer to the recreated breast.

Carcinogenic: Causing cancer

Chemotherapy: The use of strong medications to kill cancer cells.

Computer-aided detection (CAD): Artificial intelligence software used by radiologists to analyze examinations such as digital mammograms. This software highlights findings on the exam that the computer determines to be suspicious.

Core needle biopsy: A sharpened hollow tube is inserted through the skin to remove abnormal tissue for the purpose of making microscope slides for a tissue diagnosis.

Cosmetic surgery: Plastic surgery performed for purposes that are aesthetic, rather than correcting a deformity or treating a disease. Breast augmentation is an example of cosmetic surgery.

Cyst: A collection of fluid contained within a thin wall. A simple cyst contains watery fluid. A complicated cyst contains thicker fluid, has a thick wall, or may contain a mass within the fluid.

Dense breasts: Breasts that are shown on mammograms to contain more than 50 percent glandular tissue. Abnormalities can be difficult to identify on mammography if a woman has dense breasts.

Diagnostic mammogram: X-ray examination of the breast performed when a known abnormality in a woman's breast requires further workup. This abnormality could be a clinical finding, such as a palpable lump, or a mammography finding, such as calcifications found on a screening mammogram.

Digital mammography: X-ray examination of the breast performed using digital technology, rather than photographic film. A digital mammogram consists of two views of each breast.

Ductal carcinoma: Invasive breast cancer arising from the cells that line the milk ducts.

Ductal carcinoma in situ: Stage 0 breast cancer. The cancer cells are limited to the interior of the milk ducts and have not spread into the tissue surrounding the ducts.

Ectopic breast tissue: Mammary gland tissue located away from the breast.

Enzyme: Molecule that causes chemical reactions to take place in the body.

Estrogen: A female hormone important in female sexual development. Estrogen stimulates the growth of those breast cancers that possess estrogen receptors.

Excisional biopsy: Open surgery to remove abnormal tissue for the purpose of making microscope slides for a tissue diagnosis.

False positive: A medical test result that erroneously indicates that the test is abnormal, when in actuality, there is no real abnormality in the patient.

Fibrous tissue: Connective tissue consisting of collagen fibers that support many of the body's soft tissue structures.

Fine needle aspiration: Insertion of a needle through the skin to remove cells for the purpose of making microscope slides for a pathology diagnosis.

Gadolinium: A relatively safe chemical administered by intravenous injection during MRI examinations to make abnormal areas easier to detect.

Gene testing: Analysis of an individual's DNA to check for genetic abnormalities that can increase risk of genetic disease.

Gland: A body structure that secretes or excretes substances. Exocrine glands excrete liquids through ducts; for example, the mammary gland excretes milk. Endocrine glands secrete hormones into the bloodstream.

Glands of Montgomery: Sebaceous glands that form small bumps on the areola. Their function is to excrete oil that moisturizes and lubricates the nipple and areola.

HER-2 positive: Breast cancer with surface receptors for human epidermal growth factor receptor 2. HER-2 positive cancers can be treated with biologic therapy that specifically targets the cancer cells.

Hormone: A molecule released by an endocrine gland into the bloodstream to regulate body functions.

Hormone replacement therapy (HRT): The use of estrogen to treat symptoms of menopause.

Hormone therapy: The use of anti-estrogen medications to treat those breast cancers that possess estrogen receptors.

Inflammatory carcinoma: Rare form of breast cancer that causes the breast to appear red and swollen as if it is inflamed by an infection. It results from cancer cells blocking the lymph ducts of the skin of the breast.

Inframammary fold: The imaginary line at the bottom margin of the breast where the breast joins the torso.

Intraductal papilloma: Benign growth that can occur within a milk duct. It is a common cause of nipple discharge.

Introducer: A hollow metal tube slightly wider than a biopsy needle. The introducer is inserted into the breast preliminary to a needle biopsy. The biopsy needle can be inserted into the introducer multiple times to take biopsy samples from the breast.

Invasive cancer: A malignant tumor that spreads out of the duct into the surrounding tissue.

Inverted nipple: Nipple retracted below the level of the surrounding skin of the breast.

Lipoma: A benign lump composed of fat.

Lobular carcinoma: Invasive cancer that arises from the cells of the milk-producing glands that are present at the source of a milk duct.

Lobular carcinoma in situ (LCIS): Abnormal (stage 0 cancer) cells limited to the milk-producing glands that are present at the source of a milk duct.

Lumpectomy: Surgery to remove a breast cancer (and a margin of surrounding healthy tissue) while preserving the breast.

Lymph nodes: Bean-shaped structures that filter materials from the fluid in the lymph ducts.

Lymphatics: Branching ducts that carry lymph fluid through the body, removing excess fluid and foreign substances from the body.

Lymphedema: Swelling of a body part when the lymphatics are obstructed, blocking the flow of lymph fluid.

Magnetic resonance imaging (MRI): A technique for creating images of the inside of the body. The patient is placed in a strong magnetic field and scanned with radio waves.

Malignant: Cancerous

Mammary gland: The major component of the breast. The mammary gland is a modified sweat gland that makes milk.

Mammogram: An X-ray examination of the breasts.

Mass: A discrete solid growth

Mastectomy: Surgical removal of the breast

Metastasis: Cancer that has spread to a different part of the body. Plural: metastases

Milk ducts: Network of tubes that branch away from the nipple. Milk travels through these tubes to exit the mother's body and feed her infant.

Needle biopsy: Insertion of a needle through the skin to remove cells or cores of tissue for the purpose of making microscope slides for a pathology diagnosis. Techniques include fine needle aspiration, core needle biopsy, and vacuum-assisted biopsy.

Nipple discharge: Fluid that comes out of the nipple when a woman is not making milk related to pregnancy.

Nipple-sparing mastectomy: Surgery to remove the mammary gland from the breast while preserving the skin and the nipple.

Oncologist: A physician specializing in the treatment of cancer.

Oncoplastic surgery: Cancer surgery that is modified specifically to achieve an improved cosmetic result.

Probe: A handheld wand that is the part of an ultrasound machine that contacts the patient during an ultrasound examination.

Progesterone: A hormone that plays an important role in breast development and the menstrual cycle.

Prolactin: A hormone that stimulates the mammary gland to produce milk.

Prophylactic mastectomy: Removal of a healthy breast to reduce a patient's risk of future breast cancer. This is most often done for women with high risk of breast cancer, specifically carriers of BRCA gene mutations.

Radiation therapy: Use of radiation as a treatment for illness (usually cancer).

Radiologist: A physician specializing in the interpretation of medical imaging, including X-ray examinations, mammograms, CT scans, MRI examinations, and ultrasounds.

Reconstructive surgery: Surgery to correct deformity resulting from injury, previous surgery, or a birth defect. The goal of reconstructive surgery is to achieve a cosmetic result that is as close to normality as possible.

Recurrence: Cancer that returns after successful treatment of a malignancy followed by a cancer-free period.

Screening mammogram: X-ray examination of the breasts when there is no sign of a breast abnormality. A screening mammogram consists of two views of each breast, a side view and a view from above.

Sentinel lymph node biopsy: Surgical procedure to remove a small number of lymph nodes from the armpit to determine whether breast cancer has spread beyond the breast.

Solid mass: A three-dimensional lump within the breast that is not a cyst. A solid mass may be benign or malignant (cancerous).

Stereotactic biopsy: Technique for using mammogram images to guide needle biopsy of the breast.

Surgical biopsy: Open surgery to remove a block of abnormal tissue from the body for the purpose of making microscope slides for a tissue diagnosis.

Tissue expander: A tough, baglike device that is surgically placed under the skin at the mastectomy site. Over a period of weeks, saline solution (salt water) is injected through the skin into the tissue expander to gradually "inflate" the device, stretching the skin and making room for a permanent breast implant.

Ultrasound: Medical imaging technology that uses SONAR (sound waves) for creating images of structures within the body.

Vacuum-assisted biopsy: A biopsy in which a sharpened hollow tube is inserted through the skin to remove abnormal tissue for the purpose of making microscope slides for a tissue diagnosis. Cores of tissue are removed from the body using a vacuum.

X-ray technologist: Healthcare professional who takes X-ray images of patients for X-ray examinations, mammograms, and CT scans.

Resources

American Cancer Society:
Information and support services for cancer patients
800-ACS-2345
www.cancer.org

BreastCancer.org:
Information resource for breast cancer patients
610-642-6550
www.breastcancer.org

National Cancer Institute:
United States government resource for cancer information
800-4-CANCER
www.cancer.gov

NCI Cancer Genetics Services Directory:
Information relating to genetic cancer
800-4-CANCER
www.cancer.gov/about-cancer
/causes-prevention/genetics
/directory

Susan G. Komen Foundation:
Foundation for funding breast cancer research
877-GO-KOMEN
www.komen.org

Living Beyond Breast Cancer:
Support for women living with breast cancer
855-807-6386
www.lbbc.org

Radiology Information:
Information for patients regarding mammograms, breast imaging, and needle biopsies
www.radiologyinfo.org

Understanding the Mammography Screening Controversy
www.sbi-online.org
/endtheconfusion
/PatientResources.aspx

Sharsheret:
Support organization for Jewish women with breast cancer and women with BRCA mutations
866-474-2774
www.sharsheret.org

Triple Negative Breast Cancer Foundation
877-880-8622
www.tnbcfoundation.org

Bright Pink:
National organization for breast and
ovarian cancer in young women
312-787-4412
www.brightpink.org

Hope for Two:
Website for women who have cancer
while pregnant
800-743-4471
www.pregnantwithcancer.org

Save My Fertility:
Preserving fertility before and after
cancer treatment
312-503-2504
www.savemyfertility.org

Cancer Care:
Support services for cancer patients
800-813-HOPE
www.cancercare.org

Breast Cancer Trials:
Opportunities to participate in trials
of new breast cancer treatments
415-476-5777
www.breastcancertrials.org

Look Good Feel Better:
Program to help women with cancer
feel better with the help of beauty
techniques and wigs
800-395-LOOK
www.lookgoodfeelbetter.org

National Coalition for Cancer
  Survivorship
877-622-7937
www.canceradvocacy.org

Cancer Financial Assistance
  Coalition:
A coalition of organizations helping
cancer patients manage their
financial challenges
www.cancerfac.org

Cancer Support Community:
Support services for cancer patients
888-793-9355
www.cancersupportcommunity
.org

Metastatic Breast Cancer
  Network:
Advocacy organization for patients
living with metastatic breast
cancer
888-500-0370
www.mbcn.org

Bibliography

Introduction

Bates, Barbara. *A Guide to Physical Examination*, 3rd ed. Philadelphia: J.B. Lippincott Company, 1983.

Boston Women's Health Book Collective. *Our Bodies, Ourselves*. New York: Simon and Schuster, 1973.

Evers, Johannes Leonardus Henricus, and N. J. Heineman. *Gynecology: A Clinical Atlas*. St. Louis: Mosby, Inc., 1990.

Kedrowski, Karen M., and Marilyn Stine Sarow. *Cancer Activism: Gender, Media, and Public Policy*. Chicago: University of Illinois Press, 2007.

Mammography Quality Standards Act of 1992, Public Law 102-539. Congressional Record 138:3547-62. October 5, 1992.

Chapter 1: Risk Factors

Gray, Janet M., Sharima Rasanayagam, Connie Engel, and Jeanne Rizzo. "State of the Evidence 2017: An Update on the Connection Between Breast Cancer and the Environment." *Environmental Health* 16, no. 94 (2017): 1–61.

National Cancer Institute. "BRCA Mutations: Cancer Risk and Genetic Testing." www.cancer.gov/about-cancer/causes-prevention /genetics/brca-fact-sheet.

National Cancer Institute. Breast Cancer Risk Assessment Tool. https://www.cancer.gov/bcrisktool/.

Chapter 2: Breast Health Screening

American Cancer Society. "Cancer Facts and Figures 2017." https://www.cancer.org/content/dam/cancer-org/research /cancer-facts-and-statistics/annual-cancer-facts-and-figures/2017 /cancer-facts-and-figures-2017.pdf.

Hendrick, R. Edward, and Mark A. Helvie. "United States Preventive Services Task Force Screening Mammography Recommendations: Science Ignored." *American Journal of Roentgenology* 196 (2011):112–116.

Roses, Daniel F., ed. *Breast Cancer*, 2nd ed. Philadelphia: Elsevier, 2005.

Chapter 3: Mammography & Breast Imaging

Kopans, Daniel. *Breast Imaging*, 3rd ed. Philadelphia: Lippincott Williams & Wilkins, 2007.

RadiologyInfo.org for Patients. Test and Treatment Topics. https://www.radiologyinfo.org/en/submenu.cfm?pg=test-treatment.

Chapter 4: Breast Symptoms

Bennett, Barbara Bourne, Barbara G. Steinbach, N. Sisson Hardt, and Linda S. Haigh. *Breast Disease for Clinicians.* New York: McGraw-Hill, 2011.

Chapter 5: Breast Biopsy

Kuerer, Henry M., ed. *Kuerer's Breast Surgical Oncology.* New York: McGraw-Hill, 2010.

Chapter 6: Breast Cancer Facts

American Cancer Society. "Cancer Treatment and Survivorship Facts & Figures." https://www.cancer.org/research/cancer-facts-statistics /survivor-facts-figures.html.

Roses, Daniel F., ed. *Breast Cancer*, 2nd ed. Philadelphia: Elsevier, 2005.

Chapter 7: Breast Cancer Surgery

Bailey, Elizabeth. *The Patient's Checklist: 10 Simple Hospital Checklists to Keep You Safe, Sane, and Organized.* New York: Sterling Publishing Co., Inc., 2011.

Kuerer, Henry M., ed. *Kuerer's Breast Surgical Oncology.* New York: McGraw-Hill, 2010.

Chapter 8: Radiation & Medical Therapy

Kuerer, Henry M., ed. *Kuerer's Breast Surgical Oncology*. New York: McGraw-Hill, 2010.

National Comprehensive Cancer Network. *NCCN Guidelines for Treatment of Cancer by Site: Breast Cancer*. https://www.nccn.org /store/login/login.aspx?ReturnURL=https://www.nccn.org /professionals/physician_gls/pdf/breast.pdf.

Chapter 9: Reconstructive & Cosmetic Breast Surgery

Wells, Samuel A., Dorothy A. Andriole, and V. Leroy Young. *Atlas of Breast Surgery*. St. Louis: Mosby, 1994.

Picture Credits

Index

Carcinoma. *See* Breast cancer

Checklists. *See also* Breast Health Diary; *specific topics*
  about: overview and using this book, xvii–xx
  rationale for and overview of, ix–x

Chemotherapy, 93–97. *See also* Radiation treatment
  about: overview of radiation and, xx, 86; page for notes on, 98
  adjuvant chemotherapy, 94
  administering, 95
  Breast Health Diary for tracking, 154–158
  defined, **185**
  flowcharts for appropriate therapy, 96–97
  heart health and, 95–96
  how it works, 95
  neoadjuvant therapy, 94–95
  port for, 95
  preparing for treatments, 93
  to prevent recurrence of breast cancer, 94
  questions to ask if prescribed, 91
  regimens, 96–97
  side effects of, 94–95
  women over seventy and, 94

Clinical breast examination, 24–25

"Clips" (markers), biopsy, 62

Computer-aided detection (CAD), 35, 36, **185**

Contraceptives, 11

Cooper's ligaments, xiii, 46

Core needle biopsy, 59, **186**

Cosmetic breast surgery. *See also* Breast enlargement surgery; Breast reduction surgery
  about: overview of, xx, **185**; pages for notes on, 111–112
  breast lift surgery, 109
  nipple surgery, 110

Cowden syndrome, 10, 27, 39–40

Cysts
  caffeine and, 47–49
  complicated, 52
  cystic breasts, 48–49
  defined, **185**
  fibrocystic breasts, 50
  menstrual cycles and, 48, 50
  simple, 52
  size of, 48

D

DCIS. *See* Ductal carcinoma in situ (DCIS)

Density of breast, 32–34, 37–38, **185**

Diary. *See* Breast Health Diary

Dietary choices, 12. *See also* Obesity

Digital mammography, 35, 36, 38, **185**

Dimpling skin, 20, 24, 50–51

Discharge, nipple, 23, 45, **188**

Discomfort, breast, 47, 48

Doctors, contacts diary, 172–177. *See also* Oncologists; Questions to ask your doctor; Radiologists

Documenting medical facts. *See* Breast Health Diary

Ductal carcinoma, 65–66, 67–68, **185**

Ductal carcinoma in situ (DCIS)
  defined, **185**
  diagnosis, questions to ask upon, 69
  digital vs. film mammography and, 35
  mammograms detecting, 25, 31, 35, 38, 68–69
  as stage 0 breast cancer, 39, 67
  surgery saving lives, 68
  3-D mammography detecting, 38
  treating, 68–69

E

Ectopic breast tissue, xvi, **185**

Electron beam boost, 89

Enzymes, defined, **185**. *See also* Aromatase inhibitors

ERBB2 receptors, 70

Estrogen
  alcohol consumption and, 12
  blocking receptors, 6
  DCIS diagnosis and, 69
  defined, **186**
  hormone therapy, HRT and, 11, **186**
  increasing cancer risk, 6, 11
  medications to reduce, 6
  night shifts, melatonin and, 13–14
  obesity and, 13
  oral contraceptives and, 11
  ovaries and production of, 6
  receptors (ER), breast cancer and, 6, 70, 91–92. *See also* Receptors
  reducing to reduce cancer risk, 6–7

Examining your breasts. *See* Self-examination of breast

reducing tumor to avoid, 95
skin-sparing, 79–80
ultrasound exams after, 38
Medical therapy. *See also* Chemotherapy
about: definition and overview, 91; page
for notes on, 98
biologic therapy, 93, **184**
hormone therapy, 93–94, **186**
Medications
aromatase inhibitors, 6, 64–65, 92, **184**
listing, in Breast Health Diary, 160–165
risk-reducing, for BRCA gene mutations, 6
Melatonin, breast cancer and, 13–14
Men, BRCA gene mutation and breast
cancer risk, 6
Menstrual cycles. *See also* Estrogen;
Progesterone
breast discomfort and, 47
cystic breasts and, 48
fibrocystic breasts and, 50
number of, risk of breast cancer and, 14
Metastatic cancer, 67, 68, 69, 81, 86, 87, 94,
188
Milk ducts, xiii, 45, 46, 63, 66, 110, **188**
MRI, breast
about: MRI definition, **187**
additional information (website), 40
checking for multiple tumors, 40
evaluating women with newly diagnosed
cancer, 40
false positives and, 39, **186**
metal in body and, 41
preparing for, 41
results, Breast Health Diary for, 128–132
screening with, 27, 39–40
uses of, 27, 39–40
MRI-guided needle biopsies, 61–62

N

National Cancer Institute (NCI), 3, 191
National Comprehensive Cancer Network
(NCCN), 65, 86, 96–97
Needle biopsy, 56–62
about: overview of, xix
biopsy markers ("clips") for, 62
core needle biopsy, 59, **185**
defined, **188**
ease, simplicity of, 56–57
ensuring needle enters lesion, 59

fibroadenomas and, 53
fine needle aspiration, 58–59, **186**
high-risk lesion removal and, 60
image-guided, 59–62
introducers and, 62, **187**
minimally invasive, 56–57
MRI-guided, 61–62
outdated procedures compared to, 57–58
preparing for, 56
process explained, 58–62
questions to ask before, 58
results, Breast Health Diary for, 134–140
stereotactic biopsy, 62, **189**
types of, 58–59
ultrasound-guided, 60–61
vacuum-assisted, 59, **189–190**
Night shift, as risk factor, 13–14
Nipple
breast reconstruction and, 102
checking for discharge, 23
deviated or pointing away from breast at
an angle, 24
discharge, 23, 45, **188**
extra "ectopic," xvi, **185**
flaking of, 46
inverted, 24, 25, 45–46, 110, **187**
mastectomy sparing areola and, 80, **188**
Paget's disease, 46, 66
reddened or ulcerated, 24
skin changes, 46
soreness, 46, 66
structure and function, xiii–xiv
surgery, 110
symptoms, 24, 44–46

O

Obesity, 13
Oncologists, **188**
breast cancer stages used by, 66–67
doctor contacts diary, 172–177
radiation. *See* Radiation treatment
talking to regarding cancer risk, 3
Oncoplastic surgery, 75, **188**
Orange peel, skin thickening like, 23, 24, 51
Our Bodies, Ourselves, xi
Ovaries
cancer of, 5, 14
estrogen production and, 92
removal of, 6, 7, 8, 14

P

Paget's disease, 46, 66

Pain, breast, 47, 48

Patient's stories

  caffeine and breast cysts, 47–48

  cancer survivor with breast lump
    (Heather's story), 71

  family history and breast cancer (Jane's
    story), 4–5

  importance of screening mammography
    (Rosa's story), 26

Peau d'orange (skin of an orange), 23, 24, 51

Poland syndrome, xv–xvi

Pomegranate analogy, xiii

Pregnancy

  breast characteristics and, xiv

  lumps during, 51, 53

Probe, 60, **188**

Progesterone, **188**

Progesterone receptors (PR), 69, 70, 92

Prolactin, 44, **188**

Prophylactic mastectomy, 7, 8, **188**

Puberty, xv

Q

Questions to ask your doctor

  about breast cancer surgery (mastectomy,
    lumpectomy), 74

  about breast enlargement surgery, 104

  about breast lift surgery, 109

  about breast reconstruction surgery, 100

  about breast reduction surgery, 107

  about chemotherapy, 91

  about dense breasts, 34

  about needle biopsy, 58

  about radiation therapy, 87

  if diagnosed with breast cancer, 64

  if diagnosed with DCIS, 69

R

Radiation exposure, mammography and,
  34–35

Radiation treatment, 86–90. *See also*
  Chemotherapy

  about: overview of chemotherapy and,
    xx, 86; page for notes on, 98

  Breast Health Diary for tracking, 150–
    153

electron beam boost, 89

external beam radiation, 88–89

history of, for Hodgkin's lymphoma, 27, 40

how it works, 87

implanted radiation source
  (brachytherapy), 89–90, **184**

intraoperative radiation, 90

partial breast radiation options, 88, 90

questions to ask before, 87

steps in determining usefulness of, 87–88

things to have with you during, 88

uses of, 87

what to expect during, 86

Radiologists

  computer-aided detection (CAD) and,
    35, 36, **185**

  defined, 31, **189**

  doctor contacts diary, 172–177

  identifying lumpectomy target cells, 76

  MRI-guided biopsies and, 61–62

  reading mammograms, 31, 32, 36, 38

  screening vs. diagnostic mammograms
    and, 36–37

Raloxifene, 6

Receptors

  about, 70–71

  asking about DCIS diagnosis and, 69

  biologic therapy and, 93, **184**

  ERBB2, 70

  estrogen (ER), 6, 70, 91–92

  HER-2, 62, 64, 70–71, 93, 96, **186**

  hormone therapy and, 91–92, **186**

  offering unique treatment opportunity,
    70

  progesterone (PR), 69, 70, 92

Recurrence of breast cancer, 79, 80, 87, 91,
  92, 94, **189**

Resources, 191–193

Risk factors, 2–16

  about: overview of, xvii, 2–3; page for
    notes on, 16

  actions that may reduce risk of cancer, 2

  age, 10

  alcohol consumption, 11–12

  assessing your personal risk, 3

  breastfeeding reducing risk, 14

  contraceptives, 11

  controllable, 11–15

  dietary choices, 12

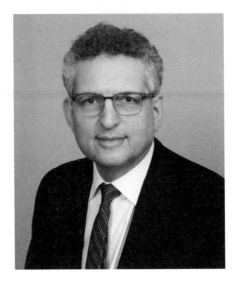

About the Author

RAND J. STACK, MD, is board certified in diagnostic radiology and has practiced in Westchester County, New York, for more than twenty-five years. He received his bachelor's degree from Yale University, his medical degree from New Jersey Medical School (now Rutgers University), and an MBA degree from Columbia University.

Dr. Stack is past president of the New York Breast Imaging Society. He is author of the chapter "Stereotactic Breast Biopsy" in the 2010 textbook *Kuerer's Breast Surgical Oncology*, and he was awarded a research grant by NYCOMED Inc. for work that he did in digital mammography. Dr. Stack has presented numerous papers at scientific meetings, is published in medical journals, and has lectured nationally.

The Breast Health Program of the Westchester County Department of Health has presented Dr. Stack with an excellence award in recognition of his service to the patients of Westchester County. In 2016, the WESTMED Medical Group presented Dr. Stack with the annual Dr. Leonard Finkelstein Excellence Award.

Dr. Stack lives in New Jersey with his wife of thirty years, Connie. They are parents of three adult children, a daughter and twin sons.